I0449198

Book design, layout, and editing by Vaughn Parker

Disclaimer:
The author, publisher, and editor of this material are not responsible in any manner whatsoever for any injury that may occur through following the instructions contained in this material. The activities, physical and otherwise, described herein are for informational purposes only. They may be too strenuous or dangerous for some people and the reader(s) should consult a physician before engaging in this or any other fitness program.

Before you start…

Don't forget to warm up!

Check out the Dynamic Flow Drills page for one of 6 possible warm-ups. These drills are meant to flow from one exercise to the next without stopping, not even when the routine calls for you to switch hands. Repeat the warm-up between 2-5 times – or until you feel you are sufficiently warmed up.

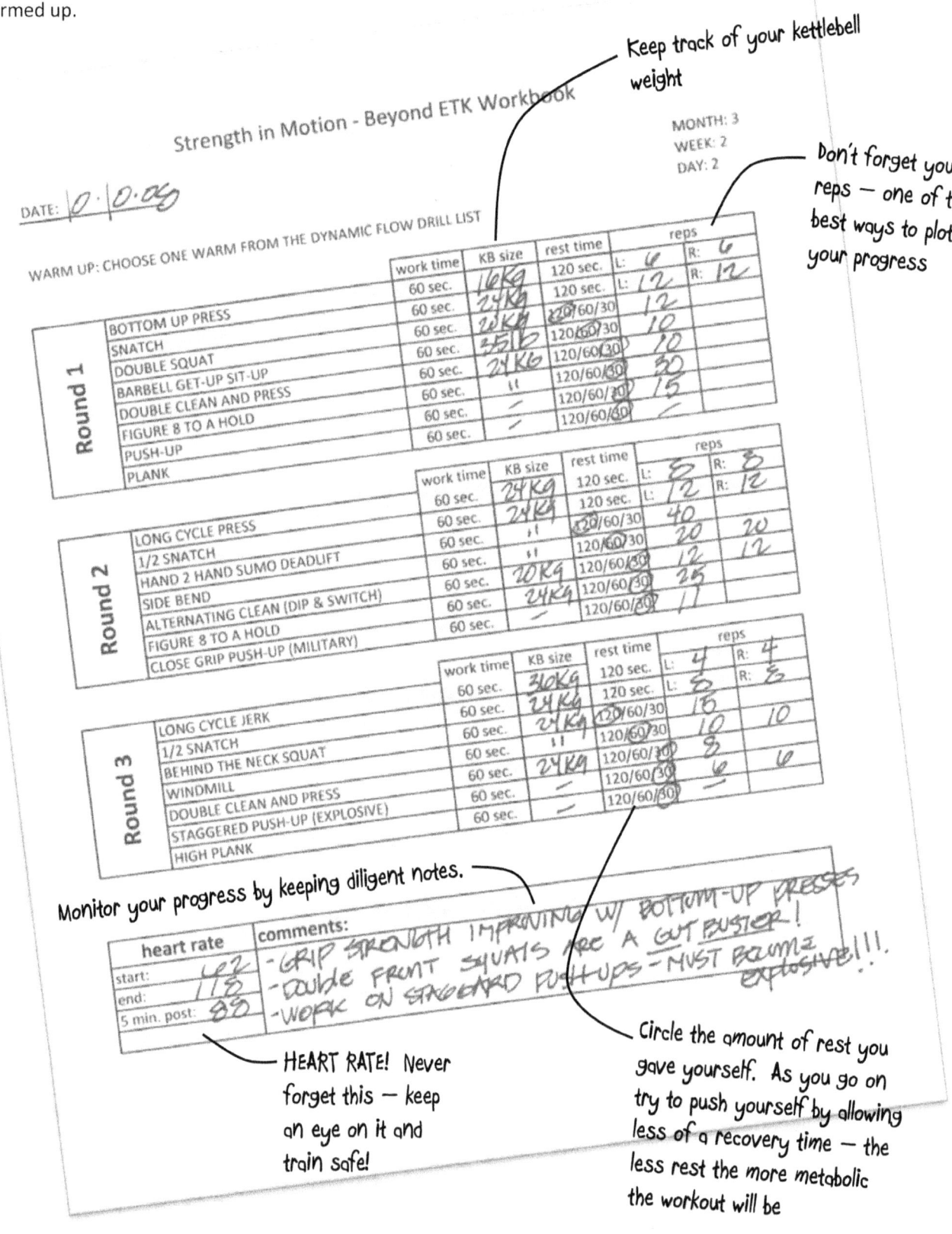

Keep track of your kettlebell weight

Strength in Motion - Beyond ETK Workbook

MONTH: 3
WEEK: 2
DAY: 2

DATE: 0·0·06

Don't forget your reps – one of the best ways to plot your progress

WARM UP: CHOOSE ONE WARM FROM THE DYNAMIC FLOW DRILL LIST

Round 1

	work time	KB size	rest time	reps	
	60 sec.	16Kg	120 sec.	L: 6	R: 6
BOTTOM UP PRESS	60 sec.	24Kg	120 sec.	L: 12	R: 12
SNATCH	60 sec.	24Kg	120/60/30	12	
DOUBLE SQUAT	60 sec.	35lb	120/60/30	10	
BARBELL GET-UP SIT-UP	60 sec.	24K6	120/60/30	10	
DOUBLE CLEAN AND PRESS	60 sec.	"	120/60/30	30	
FIGURE 8 TO A HOLD	60 sec.	—	120/60/30	15	
PUSH-UP	60 sec.		120/60/30		
PLANK					

Round 2

	work time	KB size	rest time	reps	
	60 sec.	24Kg	120 sec.	L: 8	R: 8
LONG CYCLE PRESS	60 sec.	24Kg	120 sec.	L: 12	R: 12
1/2 SNATCH	60 sec.	+1	120/60/30	40	
HAND 2 HAND SUMO DEADLIFT	60 sec.	+1	120/60/30	20	20
SIDE BEND	60 sec.	20Kg	120/60/30	12	12
ALTERNATING CLEAN (DIP & SWITCH)	60 sec.	24Kg	120/60/30	25	
FIGURE 8 TO A HOLD	60 sec.	—	120/60/30	1	
CLOSE GRIP PUSH-UP (MILITARY)					

Round 3

	work time	KB size	rest time	reps	
	60 sec.	30Kg	120 sec.	L: 4	R: 4
LONG CYCLE JERK	60 sec.	24Kg	120 sec.	L: 8	R: 8
1/2 SNATCH	60 sec.	24Kg	120/60/30	15	
BEHIND THE NECK SQUAT	60 sec.	+1	120/60/30	10	10
WINDMILL	60 sec.	24Kg	120/60/30	8	
DOUBLE CLEAN AND PRESS	60 sec.	—	120/60/30	6	6
STAGGERED PUSH-UP (EXPLOSIVE)	60 sec.	—	120/60/30		
HIGH PLANK					

Monitor your progress by keeping diligent notes.

heart rate	comments:
start: 162	- GRIP STRENGTH IMPROVING W/ BOTTOM-UP PRESSES
end: 175	- DOUBLE FRONT SQUATS ARE A GUT BUSTER!
5 min. post: 89	- WORK ON STAGGERED PUSH-UPS - MUST BECOME EXPLOSIVE!!!

HEART RATE! Never forget this – keep an eye on it and train safe!

Circle the amount of rest you gave yourself. As you go on try to push yourself by allowing less of a recovery time – the less rest the more metabolic the workout will be

Get started

That's about it. The program you are starting may well prove more physically demanding than anything you've ever attempted. Make the commitment to complete all 4 weeks before you pick up that first kettlebell. Though the volume and work performed this week will certainly be easy compared to later weeks, it may be quite a shock to the system if you are just getting started with kettlebells.

Train safe...

Im Athletic 6 Month Workout Plan

Dynamic Flow Drill Warm-ups

DFD1	repeat 2-5x
	SWINGS x10
	CLEAN AND PRESS x5
	SQUAT (KB RACKED) x5
	SNATCH x5

DFD2	repeat 2-5x
	SWINGS 10-30 L,R
	SNATCH X1 L,R
	WINDMILL X1 L,R
	TGU X1 L,R

DFD3	repeat 2-5x
	SWINGS x3
	SNATCH x3
	OVERHEAD SQUAT x3

DFD4	repeat 2-5x
	SQUAT THRUST SNATCH L,R x6 (ALT.)
	SQUAT THRUST C&P L,R x6 (ALT.)

DFD5	repeat 2-5x
	SQUAT & KICK (KB RACKED) x5 L,R
	BACK LUNGE TO PRESS x5 L,R
	FIGURE 8 TO HOLD x20 L,R

DFD6	repeat 2-5x
	1 ARM SWING 30 sec. L,R
	JUMP SQUAT 30 sec.
	HALOS 30 sec. L,R

Im Athletic 6 Month Workout Plan

DATE: _____

WARM UP: CHOOSE ONE WARM FROM THE DYNAMIC FLOW DRILL LIST

		work time	KB size	rest time	reps	
Round 1	ONE ARM PRESS	30 sec.		60 sec.	L:	R:
	1/2 SNATCH	30 sec.		60 sec.	L:	R:
	DOUBLE SQUAT	30 sec.		60/30/15		
	BARBELL GET-UP SIT-UP	30 sec.		60/30/15		
	DOUBLE KB DEAD CLEAN	30 sec.		60/30/15		
	FIGURE 8 TO A HOLD	30 sec.		60/30/15		
	PUSH-UP	30 sec.		60/30/15		
	PLANK	30 sec.		60/30/15		

		work time	KB size	rest time	reps	
Round 2	ONE ARM PUSHPRESS	30 sec.		60 sec.	L:	R:
	SNATCH	30 sec.		60 sec.	L:	R:
	HAND 2 HAND SUMO DEADLIFT	30 sec.		60/30/15		
	SIDE BEND (LEFT AND RIGHT)	30 sec.		60/30/15		
	ALTERNATING CLEAN (DIP & SWITCH)	30 sec.		60/30/15		
	FIGURE 8 TO A HOLD	30 sec.		60/30/15		
	CLOSE GRIP PUSH-UP (MILITARY)	30 sec.		60/30/15		

		work time	KB size	rest time	reps	
Round 3	LONG CYCLE JERK	30 sec.		60 sec.	L:	R:
	1/2 SNATCH	30 sec.		60 sec.	L:	R:
	BEHIND THE NECK SQUAT	30 sec.		60/30/15		
	WINDMILL (LEFT AND RIGHT)	30 sec.		60/30/15		
	DOUBLE KB LONG CYCLE CLEAN	30 sec.		60/30/15		
	STAGGERED PUSH-UP (EXPLOSIVE)	30 sec.		60/30/15		
	HIGH PLANK	30 sec.		60/30/15		

heart rate	comments:
start:	
end:	
5 min. post:	

Im Athletic 6 Month Workout Plan

WARM UP: CHOOSE ONE WARM FROM THE DYNAMIC FLOW DRILL LIST

		work time	KB size	rest time	reps	
Round 1	ONE ARM PRESS	30 sec.		60 sec.	L:	R:
	1/2 SNATCH	30 sec.		60 sec.	L:	R:
	DOUBLE SQUAT	30 sec.		60/30/15		
	BARBELL GET-UP SIT-UP	30 sec.		60/30/15		
	DOUBLE KB DEAD CLEAN	30 sec.		60/30/15		
	FIGURE 8 TO A HOLD	30 sec.		60/30/15		
	PUSH-UP	30 sec.		60/30/15		
	PLANK	30 sec.		60/30/15		

		work time	KB size	rest time	reps	
Round 2	ONE ARM PUSHPRESS	30 sec.		60 sec.	L:	R:
	SNATCH	30 sec.		60 sec.	L:	R:
	HAND 2 HAND SUMO DEADLIFT	30 sec.		60/30/15		
	SIDE BEND (LEFT AND RIGHT)	30 sec.		60/30/15		
	ALTERNATING CLEAN (DIP & SWITCH)	30 sec.		60/30/15		
	FIGURE 8 TO A HOLD	30 sec.		60/30/15		
	CLOSE GRIP PUSH-UP (MILITARY)	30 sec.		60/30/15		

		work time	KB size	rest time	reps	
Round 3	LONG CYCLE JERK	30 sec.		60 sec.	L:	R:
	1/2 SNATCH	30 sec.		60 sec.	L:	R:
	BEHIND THE NECK SQUAT	30 sec.		60/30/15		
	WINDMILL (LEFT AND RIGHT)	30 sec.		60/30/15		
	DOUBLE KB LONG CYCLE CLEAN	30 sec.		60/30/15		
	STAGGERED PUSH-UP (EXPLOSIVE)	30 sec.		60/30/15		
	HIGH PLANK	30 sec.		60/30/15		

heart rate	comments:
start:	
end:	
5 min. post:	

Im Athletic 6 Month Workout Plan

DATE: _____

WARM UP: CHOOSE ONE WARM FROM THE DYNAMIC FLOW DRILL LIST

		work time	KB size	rest time	reps	
Round 1	ONE ARM PRESS	30 sec.		60 sec.	L:	R:
	1/2 SNATCH	30 sec.		60 sec.	L:	R:
	DOUBLE SQUAT	30 sec.		60/30/15		
	BARBELL GET-UP SIT-UP	30 sec.		60/30/15		
	DOUBLE KB DEAD CLEAN	30 sec.		60/30/15		
	FIGURE 8 TO A HOLD	30 sec.		60/30/15		
	PUSH-UP	30 sec.		60/30/15		
	PLANK	30 sec.		60/30/15		

		work time	KB size	rest time	reps	
Round 2	ONE ARM PUSHPRESS	30 sec.		60 sec.	L:	R:
	SNATCH	30 sec.		60 sec.	L:	R:
	HAND 2 HAND SUMO DEADLIFT	30 sec.		60/30/15		
	SIDE BEND (LEFT AND RIGHT)	30 sec.		60/30/15		
	ALTERNATING CLEAN (DIP & SWITCH)	30 sec.		60/30/15		
	FIGURE 8 TO A HOLD	30 sec.		60/30/15		
	CLOSE GRIP PUSH-UP (MILITARY)	30 sec.		60/30/15		

		work time	KB size	rest time	reps	
Round 3	LONG CYCLE JERK	30 sec.		60 sec.	L:	R:
	1/2 SNATCH	30 sec.		60 sec.	L:	R:
	BEHIND THE NECK SQUAT	30 sec.		60/30/15		
	WINDMILL (LEFT AND RIGHT)	30 sec.		60/30/15		
	DOUBLE KB LONG CYCLE CLEAN	30 sec.		60/30/15		
	STAGGERED PUSH-UP (EXPLOSIVE)	30 sec.		60/30/15		
	HIGH PLANK	30 sec.		60/30/15		

heart rate	comments:
start:	
end:	
5 min. post:	

Im Athletic 6 Month Workout Plan

DATE: _____

WARM UP: CHOOSE ONE WARM FROM THE DYNAMIC FLOW DRILL LIST

		work time	KB size	rest time	reps	
Round 1	ONE ARM PRESS	30 sec.		60 sec.	L:	R:
	1/2 SNATCH	30 sec.		60 sec.	L:	R:
	DOUBLE SQUAT	30 sec.		60/30/15		
	BARBELL GET-UP SIT-UP	30 sec.		60/30/15		
	DOUBLE KB DEAD CLEAN	30 sec.		60/30/15		
	FIGURE 8 TO A HOLD	30 sec.		60/30/15		
	PUSH-UP	30 sec.		60/30/15		
	PLANK	30 sec.		60/30/15		

		work time	KB size	rest time	reps	
Round 2	ONE ARM PUSHPRESS	30 sec.		60 sec.	L:	R:
	SNATCH	30 sec.		60 sec.	L:	R:
	HAND 2 HAND SUMO DEADLIFT	30 sec.		60/30/15		
	SIDE BEND (LEFT AND RIGHT)	30 sec.		60/30/15		
	ALTERNATING CLEAN (DIP & SWITCH)	30 sec.		60/30/15		
	FIGURE 8 TO A HOLD	30 sec.		60/30/15		
	CLOSE GRIP PUSH-UP (MILITARY)	30 sec.		60/30/15		

		work time	KB size	rest time	reps	
Round 3	LONG CYCLE JERK	30 sec.		60 sec.	L:	R:
	1/2 SNATCH	30 sec.		60 sec.	L:	R:
	BEHIND THE NECK SQUAT	30 sec.		60/30/15		
	WINDMILL (LEFT AND RIGHT)	30 sec.		60/30/15		
	DOUBLE KB LONG CYCLE CLEAN	30 sec.		60/30/15		
	STAGGERED PUSH-UP (EXPLOSIVE)	30 sec.		60/30/15		
	HIGH PLANK	30 sec.		60/30/15		

heart rate	comments:
start:	
end:	
5 min. post:	

Im Athletic 6 Month Workout Plan

DATE: _____

WARM UP: CHOOSE ONE WARM FROM THE DYNAMIC FLOW DRILL LIST

		work time	KB size	rest time	reps	
Round 1	BOTTOM UP PRESS	30 sec.		45 sec.	L:	R:
	SNATCH	30 sec.		45 sec.	L:	R:
	DOUBLE SQUAT	30 sec.		60/30/15		
	BARBELL GET-UP SIT-UP	30 sec.		60/30/15		
	DOUBLE KB DEAD CLEAN	30 sec.		60/30/15		
	FIGURE 8 TO A HOLD	30 sec.		60/30/15		
	PUSH-UP	30 sec.		60/30/15		
	PLANK	30 sec.		60/30/15		

		work time	KB size	rest time	reps	
Round 2	LONG CYCLE PRESS	30 sec.		45 sec.	L:	R:
	1/2 SNATCH	30 sec.		45 sec.	L:	R:
	HAND 2 HAND SUMO DEADLIFT	30 sec.		60/30/15		
	SIDE BEND (LEFT AND RIGHT)	30 sec.		60/30/15		
	ALTERNATING CLEAN (DIP & SWITCH)	30 sec.		60/30/15		
	FIGURE 8 TO A HOLD	30 sec.		60/30/15		
	CLOSE GRIP PUSH-UP (MILITARY)	30 sec.		60/30/15		

		work time	KB size	rest time	reps	
Round 3	JERK	30 sec.		45 sec.	L:	R:
	SNATCH	30 sec.		45 sec.	L:	R:
	BEHIND THE NECK SQUAT	30 sec.		60/30/15		
	WINDMILL (LEFT AND RIGHT)	30 sec.		60/30/15		
	DOUBLE KB LONG CYCLE CLEAN	30 sec.		60/30/15		
	STAGGERED PUSH-UP (EXPLOSIVE)	30 sec.		60/30/15		
	HIGH PLANK	30 sec.		60/30/15		

heart rate	comments:
start:	
end:	
5 min. post:	

Im Athletic 6 Month Workout Plan

DATE: _____

WARM UP: CHOOSE ONE WARM FROM THE DYNAMIC FLOW DRILL LIST

		work time	KB size	rest time	reps	
Round 1	BOTTOM UP PRESS	30 sec.		45 sec.	L:	R:
	SNATCH	30 sec.		45 sec.	L:	R:
	DOUBLE SQUAT	30 sec.		60/30/15		
	BARBELL GET-UP SIT-UP	30 sec.		60/30/15		
	DOUBLE KB DEAD CLEAN	30 sec.		60/30/15		
	FIGURE 8 TO A HOLD	30 sec.		60/30/15		
	PUSH-UP	30 sec.		60/30/15		
	PLANK	30 sec.		60/30/15		

		work time	KB size	rest time	reps	
Round 2	LONG CYCLE PRESS	30 sec.		45 sec.	L:	R:
	1/2 SNATCH	30 sec.		45 sec.	L:	R:
	HAND 2 HAND SUMO DEADLIFT	30 sec.		60/30/15		
	SIDE BEND (LEFT AND RIGHT)	30 sec.		60/30/15		
	ALTERNATING CLEAN (DIP & SWITCH)	30 sec.		60/30/15		
	FIGURE 8 TO A HOLD	30 sec.		60/30/15		
	CLOSE GRIP PUSH-UP (MILITARY)	30 sec.		60/30/15		

		work time	KB size	rest time	reps	
Round 3	JERK	30 sec.		45 sec.	L:	R:
	SNATCH	30 sec.		45 sec.	L:	R:
	BEHIND THE NECK SQUAT	30 sec.		60/30/15		
	WINDMILL (LEFT AND RIGHT)	30 sec.		60/30/15		
	DOUBLE KB LONG CYCLE CLEAN	30 sec.		60/30/15		
	STAGGERED PUSH-UP (EXPLOSIVE)	30 sec.		60/30/15		
	HIGH PLANK	30 sec.		60/30/15		

heart rate	comments:
start:	
end:	
5 min. post:	

Im Athletic 6 Month Workout Plan

DATE: _____

WARM UP: CHOOSE ONE WARM FROM THE DYNAMIC FLOW DRILL LIST

		work time	KB size	rest time	reps	
Round 1	BOTTOM UP PRESS	30 sec.		45 sec.	L:	R:
	SNATCH	30 sec.		45 sec.	L:	R:
	DOUBLE SQUAT	30 sec.		60/30/15		
	BARBELL GET-UP SIT-UP	30 sec.		60/30/15		
	DOUBLE KB DEAD CLEAN	30 sec.		60/30/15		
	FIGURE 8 TO A HOLD	30 sec.		60/30/15		
	PUSH-UP	30 sec.		60/30/15		
	PLANK	30 sec.		60/30/15		

		work time	KB size	rest time	reps	
Round 2	LONG CYCLE PRESS	30 sec.		45 sec.	L:	R:
	1/2 SNATCH	30 sec.		45 sec.	L:	R:
	HAND 2 HAND SUMO DEADLIFT	30 sec.		60/30/15		
	SIDE BEND (LEFT AND RIGHT)	30 sec.		60/30/15		
	ALTERNATING CLEAN (DIP & SWITCH)	30 sec.		60/30/15		
	FIGURE 8 TO A HOLD	30 sec.		60/30/15		
	CLOSE GRIP PUSH-UP (MILITARY)	30 sec.		60/30/15		

		work time	KB size	rest time	reps	
Round 3	JERK	30 sec.		45 sec.	L:	R:
	SNATCH	30 sec.		45 sec.	L:	R:
	BEHIND THE NECK SQUAT	30 sec.		60/30/15		
	WINDMILL (LEFT AND RIGHT)	30 sec.		60/30/15		
	DOUBLE KB LONG CYCLE CLEAN	30 sec.		60/30/15		
	STAGGERED PUSH-UP (EXPLOSIVE)	30 sec.		60/30/15		
	HIGH PLANK	30 sec.		60/30/15		

heart rate	comments:
start:	
end:	
5 min. post:	

Im Athletic 6 Month Workout Plan

WARM UP: CHOOSE ONE WARM FROM THE DYNAMIC FLOW DRILL LIST

		work time	KB size	rest time	reps	
Round 1	BOTTOM UP PRESS	30 sec.		30 sec.	L:	R:
	SNATCH	30 sec.		30 sec.	L:	R:
	DOUBLE SQUAT	30 sec.		60/30/15		
	BARBELL GET-UP SIT-UP	30 sec.		60/30/15		
	DOUBLE KB DEAD CLEAN	30 sec.		60/30/15		
	FIGURE 8 TO A HOLD	30 sec.		60/30/15		
	PUSH-UP	30 sec.		60/30/15		
	PLANK	30 sec.		60/30/15		

		work time	KB size	rest time	reps	
Round 2	LONG CYCLE PRESS	30 sec.		30 sec.	L:	R:
	1/2 SNATCH	30 sec.		30 sec.	L:	R:
	HAND 2 HAND SUMO DEADLIFT	30 sec.		60/30/15		
	SIDE BEND (LEFT AND RIGHT)	30 sec.		60/30/15		
	ALTERNATING CLEAN (DIP & SWITCH)	30 sec.		60/30/15		
	FIGURE 8 TO A HOLD	30 sec.		60/30/15		
	CLOSE GRIP PUSH-UP (MILITARY)	30 sec.		60/30/15		

		work time	KB size	rest time	reps	
Round 3	JERK	30 sec.		30 sec.	L:	R:
	SNATCH	30 sec.		30 sec.	L:	R:
	BEHIND THE NECK SQUAT	30 sec.		60/30/15		
	WINDMILL (LEFT AND RIGHT)	30 sec.		60/30/15		
	DOUBLE KB LONG CYCLE CLEAN	30 sec.		60/30/15		
	STAGGERED PUSH-UP (EXPLOSIVE)	30 sec.		60/30/15		
	HIGH PLANK	30 sec.		60/30/15		

heart rate	comments:
start:	
end:	
5 min. post:	

Im Athletic 6 Month Workout Plan

DATE: _____

WARM UP: CHOOSE ONE WARM FROM THE DYNAMIC FLOW DRILL LIST

		work time	KB size	rest time	reps	
Round 1	LONG CYCLE JERK	30 sec.		30 sec.	L:	R:
	1/2 SNATCH	30 sec.		30 sec.	L:	R:
	DOUBLE SQUAT	30 sec.		60/30/15		
	BARBELL GET-UP SIT-UP	30 sec.		60/30/15		
	DOUBLE KB DEAD CLEAN	30 sec.		60/30/15		
	FIGURE 8 TO A HOLD	30 sec.		60/30/15		
	PUSH-UP	30 sec.		60/30/15		
	PLANK	30 sec.		60/30/15		

		work time	KB size	rest time	reps	
Round 2	JERK	30 sec.		30 sec.	L:	R:
	SNATCH	30 sec.		30 sec.	L:	R:
	HAND 2 HAND SUMO DEADLIFT	30 sec.		60/30/15		
	SIDE BEND (LEFT AND RIGHT)	30 sec.		60/30/15		
	ALTERNATING CLEAN (DIP & SWITCH)	30 sec.		60/30/15		
	FIGURE 8 TO A HOLD	30 sec.		60/30/15		
	CLOSE GRIP PUSH-UP (MILITARY)	30 sec.		60/30/15		

		work time	KB size	rest time	reps	
Round 3	BOTTOM UP PUSH PRESS	30 sec.		30 sec.	L:	R:
	1/2 SNATCH	30 sec.		30 sec.	L:	R:
	BEHIND THE NECK SQUAT	30 sec.		60/30/15		
	WINDMILL (LEFT AND RIGHT)	30 sec.		60/30/15		
	DOUBLE KB LONG CYCLE CLEAN	30 sec.		60/30/15		
	STAGGERED PUSH-UP (EXPLOSIVE)	30 sec.		60/30/15		
	HIGH PLANK	30 sec.		60/30/15		

heart rate	comments:
start:	
end:	
5 min. post:	

Im Athletic 6 Month Workout Plan

DATE: _____

WARM UP: CHOOSE ONE WARM FROM THE DYNAMIC FLOW DRILL LIST

		work time	KB size	rest time	reps	
Round 1	LONG CYCLE JERK	30 sec.		30 sec.	L:	R:
	1/2 SNATCH	30 sec.		30 sec.	L:	R:
	DOUBLE SQUAT	30 sec.		60/30/15		
	BARBELL GET-UP SIT-UP	30 sec.		60/30/15		
	DOUBLE KB DEAD CLEAN	30 sec.		60/30/15		
	FIGURE 8 TO A HOLD	30 sec.		60/30/15		
	PUSH-UP	30 sec.		60/30/15		
	PLANK	30 sec.		60/30/15		

		work time	KB size	rest time	reps	
Round 2	JERK	30 sec.		30 sec.	L:	R:
	SNATCH	30 sec.		30 sec.	L:	R:
	HAND 2 HAND SUMO DEADLIFT	30 sec.		60/30/15		
	SIDE BEND (LEFT AND RIGHT)	30 sec.		60/30/15		
	ALTERNATING CLEAN (DIP & SWITCH)	30 sec.		60/30/15		
	FIGURE 8 TO A HOLD	30 sec.		60/30/15		
	CLOSE GRIP PUSH-UP (MILITARY)	30 sec.		60/30/15		

		work time	KB size	rest time	reps	
Round 3	BOTTOM UP PUSH PRESS	30 sec.		30 sec.	L:	R:
	1/2 SNATCH	30 sec.		30 sec.	L:	R:
	BEHIND THE NECK SQUAT	30 sec.		60/30/15		
	WINDMILL (LEFT AND RIGHT)	30 sec.		60/30/15		
	DOUBLE KB LONG CYCLE CLEAN	30 sec.		60/30/15		
	STAGGERED PUSH-UP (EXPLOSIVE)	30 sec.		60/30/15		
	HIGH PLANK	30 sec.		60/30/15		

heart rate	comments:
start:	
end:	
5 min. post:	

Im Athletic 6 Month Workout Plan

DATE: _____

WARM UP: CHOOSE ONE WARM FROM THE DYNAMIC FLOW DRILL LIST

		work time	KB size	rest time	reps	
Round 1	LONG CYCLE JERK	30 sec.		30 sec.	L:	R:
	1/2 SNATCH	30 sec.		30 sec.	L:	R:
	DOUBLE SQUAT	30 sec.		60/30/15		
	BARBELL GET-UP SIT-UP	30 sec.		60/30/15		
	DOUBLE KB DEAD CLEAN	30 sec.		60/30/15		
	FIGURE 8 TO A HOLD	30 sec.		60/30/15		
	PUSH-UP	30 sec.		60/30/15		
	PLANK	30 sec.		60/30/15		

		work time	KB size	rest time	reps	
Round 2	JERK	30 sec.		30 sec.	L:	R:
	SNATCH	30 sec.		30 sec.	L:	R:
	HAND 2 HAND SUMO DEADLIFT	30 sec.		60/30/15		
	SIDE BEND (LEFT AND RIGHT)	30 sec.		60/30/15		
	ALTERNATING CLEAN (DIP & SWITCH)	30 sec.		60/30/15		
	FIGURE 8 TO A HOLD	30 sec.		60/30/15		
	CLOSE GRIP PUSH-UP (MILITARY)	30 sec.		60/30/15		

		work time	KB size	rest time	reps	
Round 3	BOTTOM UP PUSH PRESS	30 sec.		30 sec.	L:	R:
	1/2 SNATCH	30 sec.		30 sec.	L:	R:
	BEHIND THE NECK SQUAT	30 sec.		60/30/15		
	WINDMILL (LEFT AND RIGHT)	30 sec.		60/30/15		
	DOUBLE KB LONG CYCLE CLEAN	30 sec.		60/30/15		
	STAGGERED PUSH-UP (EXPLOSIVE)	30 sec.		60/30/15		
	HIGH PLANK	30 sec.		60/30/15		

heart rate	comments:
start:	
end:	
5 min. post:	

Im Athletic 6 Month Workout Plan

DATE: _____

WARM UP: CHOOSE ONE WARM FROM THE DYNAMIC FLOW DRILL LIST

Round 1		work time	KB size	rest time	reps	
	LONG CYCLE JERK	30 sec.		30 sec.	L:	R:
	1/2 SNATCH	30 sec.		30 sec.	L:	R:
	DOUBLE SQUAT	30 sec.		60/30/15		
	BARBELL GET-UP SIT-UP	30 sec.		60/30/15		
	DOUBLE KB DEAD CLEAN	30 sec.		60/30/15		
	FIGURE 8 TO A HOLD	30 sec.		60/30/15		
	PUSH-UP	30 sec.		60/30/15		
	PLANK	30 sec.		60/30/15		

Round 2		work time	KB size	rest time	reps	
	JERK	30 sec.		30 sec.	L:	R:
	SNATCH	30 sec.		30 sec.	L:	R:
	HAND 2 HAND SUMO DEADLIFT	30 sec.		60/30/15		
	SIDE BEND (LEFT AND RIGHT)	30 sec.		60/30/15		
	ALTERNATING CLEAN (DIP & SWITCH)	30 sec.		60/30/15		
	FIGURE 8 TO A HOLD	30 sec.		60/30/15		
	CLOSE GRIP PUSH-UP (MILITARY)	30 sec.		60/30/15		

Round 3		work time	KB size	rest time	reps	
	BOTTOM UP PUSH PRESS	30 sec.		30 sec.	L:	R:
	1/2 SNATCH	30 sec.		30 sec.	L:	R:
	BEHIND THE NECK SQUAT	30 sec.		60/30/15		
	WINDMILL (LEFT AND RIGHT)	30 sec.		60/30/15		
	DOUBLE KB LONG CYCLE CLEAN	30 sec.		60/30/15		
	STAGGERED PUSH-UP (EXPLOSIVE)	30 sec.		60/30/15		
	HIGH PLANK	30 sec.		60/30/15		

heart rate	comments:
start:	
end:	
5 min. post:	

Im Athletic 6 Month Workout Plan

DATE: _____

WARM UP: CHOOSE ONE WARM FROM THE DYNAMIC FLOW DRILL LIST

Round 1

	work time	KB size	rest time	reps	
PRESS	30 sec.		15 sec.	L:	R:
SNATCH	30 sec.		15 sec.	L:	R:
DOUBLE SQUAT	30 sec.		60/30/15		
BARBELL GET-UP SIT-UP	30 sec.		60/30/15		
DOUBLE KB DEAD CLEAN	30 sec.		60/30/15		
FIGURE 8 TO A HOLD	30 sec.		60/30/15		
PUSH-UP	30 sec.		60/30/15		
PLANK	30 sec.		60/30/15		

Round 2

	work time	KB size	rest time	reps	
LONG CYCLE JERK	30 sec.		15 sec.	L:	R:
SNATCH	30 sec.		15 sec.	L:	R:
HAND 2 HAND SUMO DEADLIFT	30 sec.		60/30/15		
SIDE BEND (LEFT AND RIGHT)	30 sec.		60/30/15		
ALTERNATING CLEAN (DIP & SWITCH)	30 sec.		60/30/15		
FIGURE 8 TO A HOLD	30 sec.		60/30/15		
CLOSE GRIP PUSH-UP (MILITARY)	30 sec.		60/30/15		

Round 3

	work time	KB size	rest time	reps	
JERK	30 sec.		15 sec.	L:	R:
1/2 SNATCH	30 sec.		15 sec.	L:	R:
BEHIND THE NECK SQUAT	30 sec.		60/30/15		
WINDMILL (LEFT AND RIGHT)	30 sec.		60/30/15		
DOUBLE KB LONG CYCLE CLEAN	30 sec.		60/30/15		
STAGGERED PUSH-UP (EXPLOSIVE)	30 sec.		60/30/15		
HIGH PLANK	30 sec.		60/30/15		

heart rate	comments:
start:	
end:	
5 min. post:	

Im Athletic 6 Month Workout Plan

DATE: _____

WARM UP: CHOOSE ONE WARM FROM THE DYNAMIC FLOW DRILL LIST

		work time	KB size	rest time	reps	
Round 1	PRESS	30 sec.		15 sec.	L:	R:
	SNATCH	30 sec.		15 sec.	L:	R:
	DOUBLE SQUAT	30 sec.		60/30/15		
	BARBELL GET-UP SIT-UP	30 sec.		60/30/15		
	DOUBLE KB DEAD CLEAN	30 sec.		60/30/15		
	FIGURE 8 TO A HOLD	30 sec.		60/30/15		
	PUSH-UP	30 sec.		60/30/15		
	PLANK	30 sec.		60/30/15		

		work time	KB size	rest time	reps	
Round 2	LONG CYCLE JERK	30 sec.		15 sec.	L:	R:
	SNATCH	30 sec.		15 sec.	L:	R:
	HAND 2 HAND SUMO DEADLIFT	30 sec.		60/30/15		
	SIDE BEND (LEFT AND RIGHT)	30 sec.		60/30/15		
	ALTERNATING CLEAN (DIP & SWITCH)	30 sec.		60/30/15		
	FIGURE 8 TO A HOLD	30 sec.		60/30/15		
	CLOSE GRIP PUSH-UP (MILITARY)	30 sec.		60/30/15		

		work time	KB size	rest time	reps	
Round 3	JERK	30 sec.		15 sec.	L:	R:
	1/2 SNATCH	30 sec.		15 sec.	L:	R:
	BEHIND THE NECK SQUAT	30 sec.		60/30/15		
	WINDMILL (LEFT AND RIGHT)	30 sec.		60/30/15		
	DOUBLE KB LONG CYCLE CLEAN	30 sec.		60/30/15		
	STAGGERED PUSH-UP (EXPLOSIVE)	30 sec.		60/30/15		
	HIGH PLANK	30 sec.		60/30/15		

heart rate	comments:
start:	
end:	
5 min. post:	

Im Athletic 6 Month Workout Plan

DATE: _____

WARM UP: CHOOSE ONE WARM FROM THE DYNAMIC FLOW DRILL LIST

		work time	KB size	rest time	reps	
Round 1	PRESS	30 sec.		15 sec.	L:	R:
	SNATCH	30 sec.		15 sec.	L:	R:
	DOUBLE SQUAT	30 sec.		60/30/15		
	BARBELL GET-UP SIT-UP	30 sec.		60/30/15		
	DOUBLE KB DEAD CLEAN	30 sec.		60/30/15		
	FIGURE 8 TO A HOLD	30 sec.		60/30/15		
	PUSH-UP	30 sec.		60/30/15		
	PLANK	30 sec.		60/30/15		

		work time	KB size	rest time	reps	
Round 2	LONG CYCLE JERK	30 sec.		15 sec.	L:	R:
	SNATCH	30 sec.		15 sec.	L:	R:
	HAND 2 HAND SUMO DEADLIFT	30 sec.		60/30/15		
	SIDE BEND (LEFT AND RIGHT)	30 sec.		60/30/15		
	ALTERNATING CLEAN (DIP & SWITCH)	30 sec.		60/30/15		
	FIGURE 8 TO A HOLD	30 sec.		60/30/15		
	CLOSE GRIP PUSH-UP (MILITARY)	30 sec.		60/30/15		

		work time	KB size	rest time	reps	
Round 3	JERK	30 sec.		15 sec.	L:	R:
	1/2 SNATCH	30 sec.		15 sec.	L:	R:
	BEHIND THE NECK SQUAT	30 sec.		60/30/15		
	WINDMILL (LEFT AND RIGHT)	30 sec.		60/30/15		
	DOUBLE KB LONG CYCLE CLEAN	30 sec.		60/30/15		
	STAGGERED PUSH-UP (EXPLOSIVE)	30 sec.		60/30/15		
	HIGH PLANK	30 sec.		60/30/15		

heart rate	comments:
start:	
end:	
5 min. post:	

Im Athletic 6 Month Workout Plan

DATE: _____

WARM UP: CHOOSE ONE WARM FROM THE DYNAMIC FLOW DRILL LIST

		work time	KB size	rest time	reps	
Round 1	PRESS	30 sec.		15 sec.	L:	R:
	SNATCH	30 sec.		15 sec.	L:	R:
	DOUBLE SQUAT	30 sec.		60/30/15		
	BARBELL GET-UP SIT-UP	30 sec.		60/30/15		
	DOUBLE KB DEAD CLEAN	30 sec.		60/30/15		
	FIGURE 8 TO A HOLD	30 sec.		60/30/15		
	PUSH-UP	30 sec.		60/30/15		
	PLANK	30 sec.		60/30/15		

		work time	KB size	rest time	reps	
Round 2	LONG CYCLE JERK	30 sec.		15 sec.	L:	R:
	SNATCH	30 sec.		15 sec.	L:	R:
	HAND 2 HAND SUMO DEADLIFT	30 sec.		60/30/15		
	SIDE BEND (LEFT AND RIGHT)	30 sec.		60/30/15		
	ALTERNATING CLEAN (DIP & SWITCH)	30 sec.		60/30/15		
	FIGURE 8 TO A HOLD	30 sec.		60/30/15		
	CLOSE GRIP PUSH-UP (MILITARY)	30 sec.		60/30/15		

		work time	KB size	rest time	reps	
Round 3	JERK	30 sec.		15 sec.	L:	R:
	1/2 SNATCH	30 sec.		15 sec.	L:	R:
	BEHIND THE NECK SQUAT	30 sec.		60/30/15		
	WINDMILL (LEFT AND RIGHT)	30 sec.		60/30/15		
	DOUBLE KB LONG CYCLE CLEAN	30 sec.		60/30/15		
	STAGGERED PUSH-UP (EXPLOSIVE)	30 sec.		60/30/15		
	HIGH PLANK	30 sec.		60/30/15		

heart rate	comments:
start:	
end:	
5 min. post:	

You've finished month 1!

*"**Every day you have to test yourself. If you don't, it's a wasted day.**"*
Terry Butts, Marine Corps

Im Athletic 6 Month Workout Plan

DATE: _____

WARM UP: CHOOSE ONE WARM FROM THE DYNAMIC FLOW DRILL LIST

Round 1		work time	KB size	rest time	reps	
	BOTTOM UP PRESS	45 sec.		90 sec.	L:	R:
	SNATCH	45 sec.		90 sec.	L:	R:
	DOUBLE SQUAT	30 sec.		60/30/15		
	BARBELL GET-UP SIT-UP	30 sec.		60/30/15		
	DOUBLE KB DEAD CLEAN	30 sec.		60/30/15		
	FIGURE 8 TO A HOLD	30 sec.		60/30/15		
	PUSH-UP	30 sec.		60/30/15		
	PLANK	30 sec.		60/30/15		

Round 2		work time	KB size	rest time	reps	
	ONE ARM JERK	45 sec.		90 sec.	L:	R:
	1/2 SNATCH	45 sec.		90 sec.	L:	R:
	HAND 2 HAND SUMO DEADLIFT	30 sec.		60/30/15		
	SIDE BEND (LEFT AND RIGHT)	30 sec.		60/30/15		
	ALTERNATING CLEAN (DIP & SWITCH)	30 sec.		60/30/15		
	FIGURE 8 TO A HOLD	30 sec.		60/30/15		
	CLOSE GRIP PUSH-UP (MILITARY)	30 sec.		60/30/15		

Round 3		work time	KB size	rest time	reps	
	LONG CYCLE BOTTOM UP JERK	45 sec.		90 sec.	L:	R:
	1/2 SNATCH	45 sec.		90 sec.	L:	R:
	BEHIND THE NECK SQUAT	30 sec.		60/30/15		
	WINDMILL (LEFT AND RIGHT)	30 sec.		60/30/15		
	DOUBLE KB LONG CYCLE CLEAN	30 sec.		60/30/15		
	STAGGERED PUSH-UP (EXPLOSIVE)	30 sec.		60/30/15		
	HIGH PLANK	30 sec.		60/30/15		

heart rate	comments:
start:	
end:	
5 min. post:	

Im Athletic 6 Month Workout Plan

DATE: _____

WARM UP: CHOOSE ONE WARM FROM THE DYNAMIC FLOW DRILL LIST

		work time	KB size	rest time	reps	
Round 1	BOTTOM UP PRESS	45 sec.		90 sec.	L:	R:
	SNATCH	45 sec.		90 sec.	L:	R:
	DOUBLE SQUAT	30 sec.		60/30/15		
	BARBELL GET-UP SIT-UP	30 sec.		60/30/15		
	DOUBLE KB DEAD CLEAN	30 sec.		60/30/15		
	FIGURE 8 TO A HOLD	30 sec.		60/30/15		
	PUSH-UP	30 sec.		60/30/15		
	PLANK	30 sec.		60/30/15		

		work time	KB size	rest time	reps	
Round 2	ONE ARM JERK	45 sec.		90 sec.	L:	R:
	1/2 SNATCH	45 sec.		90 sec.	L:	R:
	HAND 2 HAND SUMO DEADLIFT	30 sec.		60/30/15		
	SIDE BEND (LEFT AND RIGHT)	30 sec.		60/30/15		
	ALTERNATING CLEAN (DIP & SWITCH)	30 sec.		60/30/15		
	FIGURE 8 TO A HOLD	30 sec.		60/30/15		
	CLOSE GRIP PUSH-UP (MILITARY)	30 sec.		60/30/15		

		work time	KB size	rest time	reps	
Round 3	LONG CYCLE BOTTOM UP JERK	45 sec.		90 sec.	L:	R:
	1/2 SNATCH	45 sec.		90 sec.	L:	R:
	BEHIND THE NECK SQUAT	30 sec.		60/30/15		
	WINDMILL (LEFT AND RIGHT)	30 sec.		60/30/15		
	DOUBLE KB LONG CYCLE CLEAN	30 sec.		60/30/15		
	STAGGERED PUSH-UP (EXPLOSIVE)	30 sec.		60/30/15		
	HIGH PLANK	30 sec.		60/30/15		

heart rate	comments:
start:	
end:	
5 min. post:	

Im Athletic 6 Month Workout Plan

DATE: _____

WARM UP: CHOOSE ONE WARM FROM THE DYNAMIC FLOW DRILL LIST

Round 1		work time	KB size	rest time	reps	
	BOTTOM UP PRESS	45 sec.		90 sec.	L:	R:
	SNATCH	45 sec.		90 sec.	L:	R:
	DOUBLE SQUAT	30 sec.		60/30/15		
	BARBELL GET-UP SIT-UP	30 sec.		60/30/15		
	DOUBLE KB DEAD CLEAN	30 sec.		60/30/15		
	FIGURE 8 TO A HOLD	30 sec.		60/30/15		
	PUSH-UP	30 sec.		60/30/15		
	PLANK	30 sec.		60/30/15		

Round 2		work time	KB size	rest time	reps	
	ONE ARM JERK	45 sec.		90 sec.	L:	R:
	1/2 SNATCH	45 sec.		90 sec.	L:	R:
	HAND 2 HAND SUMO DEADLIFT	30 sec.		60/30/15		
	SIDE BEND (LEFT AND RIGHT)	30 sec.		60/30/15		
	ALTERNATING CLEAN (DIP & SWITCH)	30 sec.		60/30/15		
	FIGURE 8 TO A HOLD	30 sec.		60/30/15		
	CLOSE GRIP PUSH-UP (MILITARY)	30 sec.		60/30/15		

Round 3		work time	KB size	rest time	reps	
	LONG CYCLE BOTTOM UP JERK	45 sec.		90 sec.	L:	R:
	1/2 SNATCH	45 sec.		90 sec.	L:	R:
	BEHIND THE NECK SQUAT	30 sec.		60/30/15		
	WINDMILL (LEFT AND RIGHT)	30 sec.		60/30/15		
	DOUBLE KB LONG CYCLE CLEAN	30 sec.		60/30/15		
	STAGGERED PUSH-UP (EXPLOSIVE)	30 sec.		60/30/15		
	HIGH PLANK	30 sec.		60/30/15		

heart rate	comments:
start:	
end:	
5 min. post:	

Im Athletic 6 Month Workout Plan

DATE: _____

WARM UP: CHOOSE ONE WARM FROM THE DYNAMIC FLOW DRILL LIST

		work time	KB size	rest time	reps	
Round 1	BOTTOM UP PRESS	45 sec.		90 sec.	L:	R:
	SNATCH	45 sec.		90 sec.	L:	R:
	DOUBLE SQUAT	30 sec.		60/30/15		
	BARBELL GET-UP SIT-UP	30 sec.		60/30/15		
	DOUBLE KB DEAD CLEAN	30 sec.		60/30/15		
	FIGURE 8 TO A HOLD	30 sec.		60/30/15		
	PUSH-UP	30 sec.		60/30/15		
	PLANK	30 sec.		60/30/15		

		work time	KB size	rest time	reps	
Round 2	ONE ARM JERK	45 sec.		90 sec.	L:	R:
	1/2 SNATCH	45 sec.		90 sec.	L:	R:
	HAND 2 HAND SUMO DEADLIFT	30 sec.		60/30/15		
	SIDE BEND (LEFT AND RIGHT)	30 sec.		60/30/15		
	ALTERNATING CLEAN (DIP & SWITCH)	30 sec.		60/30/15		
	FIGURE 8 TO A HOLD	30 sec.		60/30/15		
	CLOSE GRIP PUSH-UP (MILITARY)	30 sec.		60/30/15		

		work time	KB size	rest time	reps	
Round 3	LONG CYCLE BOTTOM UP JERK	45 sec.		90 sec.	L:	R:
	1/2 SNATCH	45 sec.		90 sec.	L:	R:
	BEHIND THE NECK SQUAT	30 sec.		60/30/15		
	WINDMILL (LEFT AND RIGHT)	30 sec.		60/30/15		
	DOUBLE KB LONG CYCLE CLEAN	30 sec.		60/30/15		
	STAGGERED PUSH-UP (EXPLOSIVE)	30 sec.		60/30/15		
	HIGH PLANK	30 sec.		60/30/15		

heart rate	comments:
start:	
end:	
5 min. post:	

Im Athletic 6 Month Workout Plan

DATE: _____

WARM UP: CHOOSE ONE WARM FROM THE DYNAMIC FLOW DRILL LIST

		work time	KB size	rest time	reps	
Round 1	LONG CYCLE BOTTOM UP JERK	45 sec.		60 sec.	L:	R:
	SNATCH	45 sec.		60 sec.	L:	R:
	DOUBLE SQUAT	30 sec.		60/30/15		
	BARBELL GET-UP SIT-UP	30 sec.		60/30/15		
	DOUBLE KB DEAD CLEAN	30 sec.		60/30/15		
	FIGURE 8 TO A HOLD	30 sec.		60/30/15		
	PUSH-UP	30 sec.		60/30/15		
	PLANK	30 sec.		60/30/15		

		work time	KB size	rest time	reps	
Round 2	PRESS	45 sec.		60 sec.	L:	R:
	SNATCH	45 sec.		60 sec.	L:	R:
	HAND 2 HAND SUMO DEADLIFT	30 sec.		60/30/15		
	SIDE BEND (LEFT AND RIGHT)	30 sec.		60/30/15		
	ALTERNATING CLEAN (DIP & SWITCH)	30 sec.		60/30/15		
	FIGURE 8 TO A HOLD	30 sec.		60/30/15		
	CLOSE GRIP PUSH-UP (MILITARY)	30 sec.		60/30/15		

		work time	KB size	rest time	reps	
Round 3	JERK	45 sec.		60 sec.	L:	R:
	SNATCH	45 sec.		60 sec.	L:	R:
	BEHIND THE NECK SQUAT	30 sec.		60/30/15		
	WINDMILL (LEFT AND RIGHT)	30 sec.		60/30/15		
	DOUBLE KB LONG CYCLE CLEAN	30 sec.		60/30/15		
	STAGGERED PUSH-UP (EXPLOSIVE)	30 sec.		60/30/15		
	HIGH PLANK	30 sec.		60/30/15		

heart rate	comments:
start:	
end:	
5 min. post:	

Im Athletic 6 Month Workout Plan

DATE: _____

WARM UP: CHOOSE ONE WARM FROM THE DYNAMIC FLOW DRILL LIST

		work time	KB size	rest time	reps	
Round 1	LONG CYCLE BOTTOM UP JERK	45 sec.		60 sec.	L:	R:
	SNATCH	45 sec.		60 sec.	L:	R:
	DOUBLE SQUAT	30 sec.		60/30/15		
	BARBELL GET-UP SIT-UP	30 sec.		60/30/15		
	DOUBLE KB DEAD CLEAN	30 sec.		60/30/15		
	FIGURE 8 TO A HOLD	30 sec.		60/30/15		
	PUSH-UP	30 sec.		60/30/15		
	PLANK	30 sec.		60/30/15		

		work time	KB size	rest time	reps	
Round 2	PRESS	45 sec.		60 sec.	L:	R:
	SNATCH	45 sec.		60 sec.	L:	R:
	HAND 2 HAND SUMO DEADLIFT	30 sec.		60/30/15		
	SIDE BEND (LEFT AND RIGHT)	30 sec.		60/30/15		
	ALTERNATING CLEAN (DIP & SWITCH)	30 sec.		60/30/15		
	FIGURE 8 TO A HOLD	30 sec.		60/30/15		
	CLOSE GRIP PUSH-UP (MILITARY)	30 sec.		60/30/15		

		work time	KB size	rest time	reps	
Round 3	JERK	45 sec.		60 sec.	L:	R:
	SNATCH	45 sec.		60 sec.	L:	R:
	BEHIND THE NECK SQUAT	30 sec.		60/30/15		
	WINDMILL (LEFT AND RIGHT)	30 sec.		60/30/15		
	DOUBLE KB LONG CYCLE CLEAN	30 sec.		60/30/15		
	STAGGERED PUSH-UP (EXPLOSIVE)	30 sec.		60/30/15		
	HIGH PLANK	30 sec.		60/30/15		

heart rate	comments:
start:	
end:	
5 min. post:	

Im Athletic 6 Month Workout Plan

DATE: _____

WARM UP: CHOOSE ONE WARM FROM THE DYNAMIC FLOW DRILL LIST

		work time	KB size	rest time	reps	
Round 1	LONG CYCLE BOTTOM UP JERK	45 sec.		60 sec.	L:	R:
	SNATCH	45 sec.		60 sec.	L:	R:
	DOUBLE SQUAT	30 sec.		60/30/15		
	BARBELL GET-UP SIT-UP	30 sec.		60/30/15		
	DOUBLE KB DEAD CLEAN	30 sec.		60/30/15		
	FIGURE 8 TO A HOLD	30 sec.		60/30/15		
	PUSH-UP	30 sec.		60/30/15		
	PLANK	30 sec.		60/30/15		

		work time	KB size	rest time	reps	
Round 2	PRESS	45 sec.		60 sec.	L:	R:
	SNATCH	45 sec.		60 sec.	L:	R:
	HAND 2 HAND SUMO DEADLIFT	30 sec.		60/30/15		
	SIDE BEND (LEFT AND RIGHT)	30 sec.		60/30/15		
	ALTERNATING CLEAN (DIP & SWITCH)	30 sec.		60/30/15		
	FIGURE 8 TO A HOLD	30 sec.		60/30/15		
	CLOSE GRIP PUSH-UP (MILITARY)	30 sec.		60/30/15		

		work time	KB size	rest time	reps	
Round 3	JERK	45 sec.		60 sec.	L:	R:
	SNATCH	45 sec.		60 sec.	L:	R:
	BEHIND THE NECK SQUAT	30 sec.		60/30/15		
	WINDMILL (LEFT AND RIGHT)	30 sec.		60/30/15		
	DOUBLE KB LONG CYCLE CLEAN	30 sec.		60/30/15		
	STAGGERED PUSH-UP (EXPLOSIVE)	30 sec.		60/30/15		
	HIGH PLANK	30 sec.		60/30/15		

heart rate	comments:
start:	
end:	
5 min. post:	

Im Athletic 6 Month Workout Plan

DATE: _____

WARM UP: CHOOSE ONE WARM FROM THE DYNAMIC FLOW DRILL LIST

		work time	KB size	rest time	reps	
Round 1	LONG CYCLE BOTTOM UP JERK	45 sec.		60 sec.	L:	R:
	SNATCH	45 sec.		60 sec.	L:	R:
	DOUBLE SQUAT	30 sec.		60/30/15		
	BARBELL GET-UP SIT-UP	30 sec.		60/30/15		
	DOUBLE KB DEAD CLEAN	30 sec.		60/30/15		
	FIGURE 8 TO A HOLD	30 sec.		60/30/15		
	PUSH-UP	30 sec.		60/30/15		
	PLANK	30 sec.		60/30/15		

		work time	KB size	rest time	reps	
Round 2	PRESS	45 sec.		60 sec.	L:	R:
	SNATCH	45 sec.		60 sec.	L:	R:
	HAND 2 HAND SUMO DEADLIFT	30 sec.		60/30/15		
	SIDE BEND (LEFT AND RIGHT)	30 sec.		60/30/15		
	ALTERNATING CLEAN (DIP & SWITCH)	30 sec.		60/30/15		
	FIGURE 8 TO A HOLD	30 sec.		60/30/15		
	CLOSE GRIP PUSH-UP (MILITARY)	30 sec.		60/30/15		

		work time	KB size	rest time	reps	
Round 3	JERK	45 sec.		60 sec.	L:	R:
	SNATCH	45 sec.		60 sec.	L:	R:
	BEHIND THE NECK SQUAT	30 sec.		60/30/15		
	WINDMILL (LEFT AND RIGHT)	30 sec.		60/30/15		
	DOUBLE KB LONG CYCLE CLEAN	30 sec.		60/30/15		
	STAGGERED PUSH-UP (EXPLOSIVE)	30 sec.		60/30/15		
	HIGH PLANK	30 sec.		60/30/15		

heart rate	comments:
start:	
end:	
5 min. post:	

Im Athletic 6 Month Workout Plan

DATE: _____

WARM UP: CHOOSE ONE WARM FROM THE DYNAMIC FLOW DRILL LIST

Round 1

	work time	KB size	rest time	reps	
LONG CYCLE JERK	45 sec.		40 sec.	L:	R:
1/2 SNATCH	45 sec.		40 sec.	L:	R:
DOUBLE SQUAT	30 sec.		60/30/15		
BARBELL GET-UP SIT-UP	30 sec.		60/30/15		
DOUBLE KB DEAD CLEAN	30 sec.		60/30/15		
FIGURE 8 TO A HOLD	30 sec.		60/30/15		
PUSH-UP	30 sec.		60/30/15		
PLANK	30 sec.		60/30/15		

Round 2

	work time	KB size	rest time	reps	
LONG CYCLE PRESS	45 sec.		40 sec.	L:	R:
1/2 SNATCH	45 sec.		40 sec.	L:	R:
HAND 2 HAND SUMO DEADLIFT	30 sec.		60/30/15		
SIDE BEND (LEFT AND RIGHT)	30 sec.		60/30/15		
ALTERNATING CLEAN (DIP & SWITCH)	30 sec.		60/30/15		
FIGURE 8 TO A HOLD	30 sec.		60/30/15		
CLOSE GRIP PUSH-UP (MILITARY)	30 sec.		60/30/15		

Round 3

	work time	KB size	rest time	reps	
JERK	45 sec.		40 sec.	L:	R:
1/2 SNATCH	45 sec.		40 sec.	L:	R:
BEHIND THE NECK SQUAT	30 sec.		60/30/15		
WINDMILL (LEFT AND RIGHT)	30 sec.		60/30/15		
DOUBLE KB LONG CYCLE CLEAN	30 sec.		60/30/15		
STAGGERED PUSH-UP (EXPLOSIVE)	30 sec.		60/30/15		
HIGH PLANK	30 sec.		60/30/15		

heart rate	comments:
start:	
end:	
5 min. post:	

Im Athletic 6 Month Workout Plan

DATE: _____

MONTH: 2
WEEK: 3
DAY: 2

WARM UP: CHOOSE ONE WARM FROM THE DYNAMIC FLOW DRILL LIST

		work time	KB size	rest time	reps	
Round 1	LONG CYCLE JERK	45 sec.		40 sec.	L:	R:
	1/2 SNATCH	45 sec.		40 sec.	L:	R:
	DOUBLE SQUAT	30 sec.		60/30/15		
	BARBELL GET-UP SIT-UP	30 sec.		60/30/15		
	DOUBLE KB DEAD CLEAN	30 sec.		60/30/15		
	FIGURE 8 TO A HOLD	30 sec.		60/30/15		
	PUSH-UP	30 sec.		60/30/15		
	PLANK	30 sec.		60/30/15		

		work time	KB size	rest time	reps	
Round 2	LONG CYCLE PRESS	45 sec.		40 sec.	L:	R:
	1/2 SNATCH	45 sec.		40 sec.	L:	R:
	HAND 2 HAND SUMO DEADLIFT	30 sec.		60/30/15		
	SIDE BEND (LEFT AND RIGHT)	30 sec.		60/30/15		
	ALTERNATING CLEAN (DIP & SWITCH)	30 sec.		60/30/15		
	FIGURE 8 TO A HOLD	30 sec.		60/30/15		
	CLOSE GRIP PUSH-UP (MILITARY)	30 sec.		60/30/15		

		work time	KB size	rest time	reps	
Round 3	JERK	45 sec.		40 sec.	L:	R:
	1/2 SNATCH	45 sec.		40 sec.	L:	R:
	BEHIND THE NECK SQUAT	30 sec.		60/30/15		
	WINDMILL (LEFT AND RIGHT)	30 sec.		60/30/15		
	DOUBLE KB LONG CYCLE CLEAN	30 sec.		60/30/15		
	STAGGERED PUSH-UP (EXPLOSIVE)	30 sec.		60/30/15		
	HIGH PLANK	30 sec.		60/30/15		

heart rate	comments:
start:	
end:	
5 min. post:	

Im Athletic 6 Month Workout Plan

DATE: _____

MONTH: 2
WEEK: 3
DAY: 3

WARM UP: CHOOSE ONE WARM FROM THE DYNAMIC FLOW DRILL LIST

		work time	KB size	rest time	reps	
Round 1	LONG CYCLE JERK	45 sec.		40 sec.	L:	R:
	1/2 SNATCH	45 sec.		40 sec.	L:	R:
	DOUBLE SQUAT	30 sec.		60/30/15		
	BARBELL GET-UP SIT-UP	30 sec.		60/30/15		
	DOUBLE KB DEAD CLEAN	30 sec.		60/30/15		
	FIGURE 8 TO A HOLD	30 sec.		60/30/15		
	PUSH-UP	30 sec.		60/30/15		
	PLANK	30 sec.		60/30/15		

		work time	KB size	rest time	reps	
Round 2	LONG CYCLE PRESS	45 sec.		40 sec.	L:	R:
	1/2 SNATCH	45 sec.		40 sec.	L:	R:
	HAND 2 HAND SUMO DEADLIFT	30 sec.		60/30/15		
	SIDE BEND (LEFT AND RIGHT)	30 sec.		60/30/15		
	ALTERNATING CLEAN (DIP & SWITCH)	30 sec.		60/30/15		
	FIGURE 8 TO A HOLD	30 sec.		60/30/15		
	CLOSE GRIP PUSH-UP (MILITARY)	30 sec.		60/30/15		

		work time	KB size	rest time	reps	
Round 3	JERK	45 sec.		40 sec.	L:	R:
	1/2 SNATCH	45 sec.		40 sec.	L:	R:
	BEHIND THE NECK SQUAT	30 sec.		60/30/15		
	WINDMILL (LEFT AND RIGHT)	30 sec.		60/30/15		
	DOUBLE KB LONG CYCLE CLEAN	30 sec.		60/30/15		
	STAGGERED PUSH-UP (EXPLOSIVE)	30 sec.		60/30/15		
	HIGH PLANK	30 sec.		60/30/15		

heart rate	comments:
start:	
end:	
5 min. post:	

Im Athletic 6 Month Workout Plan

DATE: _____

WARM UP: CHOOSE ONE WARM FROM THE DYNAMIC FLOW DRILL LIST

		work time	KB size	rest time	reps	
Round 1	LONG CYCLE JERK	45 sec.		40 sec.	L:	R:
	1/2 SNATCH	45 sec.		40 sec.	L:	R:
	DOUBLE SQUAT	30 sec.		60/30/15		
	BARBELL GET-UP SIT-UP	30 sec.		60/30/15		
	DOUBLE KB DEAD CLEAN	30 sec.		60/30/15		
	FIGURE 8 TO A HOLD	30 sec.		60/30/15		
	PUSH-UP	30 sec.		60/30/15		
	PLANK	30 sec.		60/30/15		

		work time	KB size	rest time	reps	
Round 2	LONG CYCLE PRESS	45 sec.		40 sec.	L:	R:
	1/2 SNATCH	45 sec.		40 sec.	L:	R:
	HAND 2 HAND SUMO DEADLIFT	30 sec.		60/30/15		
	SIDE BEND (LEFT AND RIGHT)	30 sec.		60/30/15		
	ALTERNATING CLEAN (DIP & SWITCH)	30 sec.		60/30/15		
	FIGURE 8 TO A HOLD	30 sec.		60/30/15		
	CLOSE GRIP PUSH-UP (MILITARY)	30 sec.		60/30/15		

		work time	KB size	rest time	reps	
Round 3	JERK	45 sec.		40 sec.	L:	R:
	1/2 SNATCH	45 sec.		40 sec.	L:	R:
	BEHIND THE NECK SQUAT	30 sec.		60/30/15		
	WINDMILL (LEFT AND RIGHT)	30 sec.		60/30/15		
	DOUBLE KB LONG CYCLE CLEAN	30 sec.		60/30/15		
	STAGGERED PUSH-UP (EXPLOSIVE)	30 sec.		60/30/15		
	HIGH PLANK	30 sec.		60/30/15		

heart rate	comments:
start:	
end:	
5 min. post:	

Im Athletic 6 Month Workout Plan

WARM UP: CHOOSE ONE WARM FROM THE DYNAMIC FLOW DRILL LIST

Round 1

	work time	KB size	rest time	reps	
PUSH PRESS	45 sec.		20 sec.	L:	R:
SNATCH	45 sec.		20 sec.	L:	R:
DOUBLE SQUAT	30 sec.		60/30/15		
BARBELL GET-UP SIT-UP	30 sec.		60/30/15		
DOUBLE KB DEAD CLEAN	30 sec.		60/30/15		
FIGURE 8 TO A HOLD	30 sec.		60/30/15		
PUSH-UP	30 sec.		60/30/15		
PLANK	30 sec.		60/30/15		

Round 2

	work time	KB size	rest time	reps	
LONG CYCLE PRESS	45 sec.		20 sec.	L:	R:
1/2 SNATCH	45 sec.		20 sec.	L:	R:
HAND 2 HAND SUMO DEADLIFT	30 sec.		60/30/15		
SIDE BEND (LEFT AND RIGHT)	30 sec.		60/30/15		
ALTERNATING CLEAN (DIP & SWITCH)	30 sec.		60/30/15		
FIGURE 8 TO A HOLD	30 sec.		60/30/15		
CLOSE GRIP PUSH-UP (MILITARY)	30 sec.		60/30/15		

Round 3

	work time	KB size	rest time	reps	
LONG CYCLE BOTTOM UP PRESS	45 sec.		20 sec.	L:	R:
1/2 SNATCH	45 sec.		20 sec.	L:	R:
BEHIND THE NECK SQUAT	30 sec.		60/30/15		
WINDMILL (LEFT AND RIGHT)	30 sec.		60/30/15		
DOUBLE KB LONG CYCLE CLEAN	30 sec.		60/30/15		
STAGGERED PUSH-UP (EXPLOSIVE)	30 sec.		60/30/15		
HIGH PLANK	30 sec.		60/30/15		

heart rate	comments:
start:	
end:	
5 min. post:	

Im Athletic 6 Month Workout Plan

DATE: _____

WARM UP: CHOOSE ONE WARM FROM THE DYNAMIC FLOW DRILL LIST

		work time	KB size	rest time	reps	
Round 1	PUSH PRESS	45 sec.		20 sec.	L:	R:
	SNATCH	45 sec.		20 sec.	L:	R:
	DOUBLE SQUAT	30 sec.		60/30/15		
	BARBELL GET-UP SIT-UP	30 sec.		60/30/15		
	DOUBLE KB DEAD CLEAN	30 sec.		60/30/15		
	FIGURE 8 TO A HOLD	30 sec.		60/30/15		
	PUSH-UP	30 sec.		60/30/15		
	PLANK	30 sec.		60/30/15		

		work time	KB size	rest time	reps	
Round 2	LONG CYCLE PRESS	45 sec.		20 sec.	L:	R:
	1/2 SNATCH	45 sec.		20 sec.	L:	R:
	HAND 2 HAND SUMO DEADLIFT	30 sec.		60/30/15		
	SIDE BEND (LEFT AND RIGHT)	30 sec.		60/30/15		
	ALTERNATING CLEAN (DIP & SWITCH)	30 sec.		60/30/15		
	FIGURE 8 TO A HOLD	30 sec.		60/30/15		
	CLOSE GRIP PUSH-UP (MILITARY)	30 sec.		60/30/15		

		work time	KB size	rest time	reps	
Round 3	LONG CYCLE BOTTOM UP PRESS	45 sec.		20 sec.	L:	R:
	1/2 SNATCH	45 sec.		20 sec.	L:	R:
	BEHIND THE NECK SQUAT	30 sec.		60/30/15		
	WINDMILL (LEFT AND RIGHT)	30 sec.		60/30/15		
	DOUBLE KB LONG CYCLE CLEAN	30 sec.		60/30/15		
	STAGGERED PUSH-UP (EXPLOSIVE)	30 sec.		60/30/15		
	HIGH PLANK	30 sec.		60/30/15		

heart rate	comments:
start:	
end:	
5 min. post:	

Strength in Motion - Beyond ETK Workbook

DATE: _____

MONTH: 2
WEEK: 4
DAY: 3

WARM UP: CHOOSE ONE WARM FROM THE DYNAMIC FLOW DRILL LIST

		work time	KB size	rest time	reps	
Round 1	PUSH PRESS	45 sec.		20 sec.	L:	R:
	SNATCH	45 sec.		20 sec.	L:	R:
	DOUBLE SQUAT	30 sec.		60/30/15		
	BARBELL GET-UP SIT-UP	30 sec.		60/30/15		
	DOUBLE KB DEAD CLEAN	30 sec.		60/30/15		
	FIGURE 8 TO A HOLD	30 sec.		60/30/15		
	PUSH-UP	30 sec.		60/30/15		
	PLANK	30 sec.		60/30/15		

		work time	KB size	rest time	reps	
Round 2	LONG CYCLE PRESS	45 sec.		20 sec.	L:	R:
	1/2 SNATCH	45 sec.		20 sec.	L:	R:
	HAND 2 HAND SUMO DEADLIFT	30 sec.		60/30/15		
	SIDE BEND (LEFT AND RIGHT)	30 sec.		60/30/15		
	ALTERNATING CLEAN (DIP & SWITCH)	30 sec.		60/30/15		
	FIGURE 8 TO A HOLD	30 sec.		60/30/15		
	CLOSE GRIP PUSH-UP (MILITARY)	30 sec.		60/30/15		

		work time	KB size	rest time	reps	
Round 3	LONG CYCLE BOTTOM UP PRESS	45 sec.		20 sec.	L:	R:
	1/2 SNATCH	45 sec.		20 sec.	L:	R:
	BEHIND THE NECK SQUAT	30 sec.		60/30/15		
	WINDMILL (LEFT AND RIGHT)	30 sec.		60/30/15		
	DOUBLE KB LONG CYCLE CLEAN	30 sec.		60/30/15		
	STAGGERED PUSH-UP (EXPLOSIVE)	30 sec.		60/30/15		
	HIGH PLANK	30 sec.		60/30/15		

heart rate	comments:
start:	
end:	
5 min. post:	

Im Athletic 6 Month Workout Plan

DATE: _____

WARM UP: CHOOSE ONE WARM FROM THE DYNAMIC FLOW DRILL LIST

Round 1

	work time	KB size	rest time	reps	
PUSH PRESS	45 sec.		20 sec.	L:	R:
SNATCH	45 sec.		20 sec.	L:	R:
DOUBLE SQUAT	30 sec.		60/30/15		
BARBELL GET-UP SIT-UP	30 sec.		60/30/15		
DOUBLE KB DEAD CLEAN	30 sec.		60/30/15		
FIGURE 8 TO A HOLD	30 sec.		60/30/15		
PUSH-UP	30 sec.		60/30/15		
PLANK	30 sec.		60/30/15		

Round 2

	work time	KB size	rest time	reps	
LONG CYCLE PRESS	45 sec.		20 sec.	L:	R:
1/2 SNATCH	45 sec.		20 sec.	L:	R:
HAND 2 HAND SUMO DEADLIFT	30 sec.		60/30/15		
SIDE BEND (LEFT AND RIGHT)	30 sec.		60/30/15		
ALTERNATING CLEAN (DIP & SWITCH)	30 sec.		60/30/15		
FIGURE 8 TO A HOLD	30 sec.		60/30/15		
CLOSE GRIP PUSH-UP (MILITARY)	30 sec.		60/30/15		

Round 3

	work time	KB size	rest time	reps	
LONG CYCLE BOTTOM UP PRESS	45 sec.		20 sec.	L:	R:
1/2 SNATCH	45 sec.		20 sec.	L:	R:
BEHIND THE NECK SQUAT	30 sec.		60/30/15		
WINDMILL (LEFT AND RIGHT)	30 sec.		60/30/15		
DOUBLE KB LONG CYCLE CLEAN	30 sec.		60/30/15		
STAGGERED PUSH-UP (EXPLOSIVE)	30 sec.		60/30/15		
HIGH PLANK	30 sec.		60/30/15		

heart rate	comments:
start:	
end:	
5 min. post:	

You've finished month 2!

Benefit No. 1 to Kettlebell training:

Burns Fat in Less Time: Kettlebell training by its nature is metabolic, that is, it's based in cardio all while giving you the benefit of a strength training workout. Most of our workouts are performed "circuit style" with little to no break between rounds - offering maximum calorie burn in excess of 800-1000 calories for every 45-60 minute workout. That means no more stair stepper...

Im Athletic 6 Month Workout Plan

DATE: _____

WARM UP: CHOOSE ONE WARM FROM THE DYNAMIC FLOW DRILL LIST

		work time	KB size	rest time	reps	
Round 1	BOTTOM UP JERK	60 sec.		120 sec.	L:	R:
	1/2 SNATCH	60 sec.		120 sec.	L:	R:
	DOUBLE SQUAT	30 sec.		60/30/15		
	BARBELL GET-UP SIT-UP	30 sec.		60/30/15		
	DOUBLE KB DEAD CLEAN	30 sec.		60/30/15		
	FIGURE 8 TO A HOLD	30 sec.		60/30/15		
	PUSH-UP	30 sec.		60/30/15		
	PLANK	30 sec.		60/30/15		

		work time	KB size	rest time	reps	
Round 2	LONG CYCLE JERK	60 sec.		120 sec.	L:	R:
	1/2 SNATCH	60 sec.		120 sec.	L:	R:
	HAND 2 HAND SUMO DEADLIFT	30 sec.		60/30/15		
	SIDE BEND (LEFT AND RIGHT)	30 sec.		60/30/15		
	ALTERNATING CLEAN (DIP & SWITCH)	30 sec.		60/30/15		
	FIGURE 8 TO A HOLD	30 sec.		60/30/15		
	CLOSE GRIP PUSH-UP (MILITARY)	30 sec.		60/30/15		

		work time	KB size	rest time	reps	
Round 3	JERK	60 sec.		120 sec.	L:	R:
	SNATCH	60 sec.		120 sec.	L:	R:
	BEHIND THE NECK SQUAT	30 sec.		60/30/15		
	WINDMILL (LEFT AND RIGHT)	30 sec.		60/30/15		
	DOUBLE KB LONG CYCLE CLEAN	30 sec.		60/30/15		
	STAGGERED PUSH-UP (EXPLOSIVE)	30 sec.		60/30/15		
	HIGH PLANK	30 sec.		60/30/15		

heart rate	comments:
start:	
end:	
5 min. post:	

Im Athletic 6 Month Workout Plan

DATE: _____

MONTH: 3
WEEK: 1
DAY: 2

WARM UP: CHOOSE ONE WARM FROM THE DYNAMIC FLOW DRILL LIST

		work time	KB size	rest time	reps	
Round 1	BOTTOM UP JERK	60 sec.		120 sec.	L:	R:
	1/2 SNATCH	60 sec.		120 sec.	L:	R:
	DOUBLE SQUAT	30 sec.		60/30/15		
	BARBELL GET-UP SIT-UP	30 sec.		60/30/15		
	DOUBLE KB DEAD CLEAN	30 sec.		60/30/15		
	FIGURE 8 TO A HOLD	30 sec.		60/30/15		
	PUSH-UP	30 sec.		60/30/15		
	PLANK	30 sec.		60/30/15		

		work time	KB size	rest time	reps	
Round 2	LONG CYCLE JERK	60 sec.		120 sec.	L:	R:
	1/2 SNATCH	60 sec.		120 sec.	L:	R:
	HAND 2 HAND SUMO DEADLIFT	30 sec.		60/30/15		
	SIDE BEND (LEFT AND RIGHT)	30 sec.		60/30/15		
	ALTERNATING CLEAN (DIP & SWITCH)	30 sec.		60/30/15		
	FIGURE 8 TO A HOLD	30 sec.		60/30/15		
	CLOSE GRIP PUSH-UP (MILITARY)	30 sec.		60/30/15		

		work time	KB size	rest time	reps	
Round 3	JERK	60 sec.		120 sec.	L:	R:
	SNATCH	60 sec.		120 sec.	L:	R:
	BEHIND THE NECK SQUAT	30 sec.		60/30/15		
	WINDMILL (LEFT AND RIGHT)	30 sec.		60/30/15		
	DOUBLE KB LONG CYCLE CLEAN	30 sec.		60/30/15		
	STAGGERED PUSH-UP (EXPLOSIVE)	30 sec.		60/30/15		
	HIGH PLANK	30 sec.		60/30/15		

heart rate	comments:
start:	
end:	
5 min. post:	

Im Athletic 6 Month Workout Plan

DATE: _____

WARM UP: CHOOSE ONE WARM FROM THE DYNAMIC FLOW DRILL LIST

		work time	KB size	rest time	reps	
Round 1	BOTTOM UP JERK	60 sec.		120 sec.	L:	R:
	1/2 SNATCH	60 sec.		120 sec.	L:	R:
	DOUBLE SQUAT	30 sec.		60/30/15		
	BARBELL GET-UP SIT-UP	30 sec.		60/30/15		
	DOUBLE KB DEAD CLEAN	30 sec.		60/30/15		
	FIGURE 8 TO A HOLD	30 sec.		60/30/15		
	PUSH-UP	30 sec.		60/30/15		
	PLANK	30 sec.		60/30/15		

		work time	KB size	rest time	reps	
Round 2	LONG CYCLE JERK	60 sec.		120 sec.	L:	R:
	1/2 SNATCH	60 sec.		120 sec.	L:	R:
	HAND 2 HAND SUMO DEADLIFT	30 sec.		60/30/15		
	SIDE BEND (LEFT AND RIGHT)	30 sec.		60/30/15		
	ALTERNATING CLEAN (DIP & SWITCH)	30 sec.		60/30/15		
	FIGURE 8 TO A HOLD	30 sec.		60/30/15		
	CLOSE GRIP PUSH-UP (MILITARY)	30 sec.		60/30/15		

		work time	KB size	rest time	reps	
Round 3	JERK	60 sec.		120 sec.	L:	R:
	SNATCH	60 sec.		120 sec.	L:	R:
	BEHIND THE NECK SQUAT	30 sec.		60/30/15		
	WINDMILL (LEFT AND RIGHT)	30 sec.		60/30/15		
	DOUBLE KB LONG CYCLE CLEAN	30 sec.		60/30/15		
	STAGGERED PUSH-UP (EXPLOSIVE)	30 sec.		60/30/15		
	HIGH PLANK	30 sec.		60/30/15		

heart rate	comments:
start:	
end:	
5 min. post:	

Im Athletic 6 Month Workout Plan

DATE: _____

WARM UP: CHOOSE ONE WARM FROM THE DYNAMIC FLOW DRILL LIST

		work time	KB size	rest time	reps	
Round 1	BOTTOM UP JERK	60 sec.		120 sec.	L:	R:
	1/2 SNATCH	60 sec.		120 sec.	L:	R:
	DOUBLE SQUAT	30 sec.		60/30/15		
	BARBELL GET-UP SIT-UP	30 sec.		60/30/15		
	DOUBLE KB DEAD CLEAN	30 sec.		60/30/15		
	FIGURE 8 TO A HOLD	30 sec.		60/30/15		
	PUSH-UP	30 sec.		60/30/15		
	PLANK	30 sec.		60/30/15		

		work time	KB size	rest time	reps	
Round 2	LONG CYCLE JERK	60 sec.		120 sec.	L:	R:
	1/2 SNATCH	60 sec.		120 sec.	L:	R:
	HAND 2 HAND SUMO DEADLIFT	30 sec.		60/30/15		
	SIDE BEND (LEFT AND RIGHT)	30 sec.		60/30/15		
	ALTERNATING CLEAN (DIP & SWITCH)	30 sec.		60/30/15		
	FIGURE 8 TO A HOLD	30 sec.		60/30/15		
	CLOSE GRIP PUSH-UP (MILITARY)	30 sec.		60/30/15		

		work time	KB size	rest time	reps	
Round 3	JERK	60 sec.		120 sec.	L:	R:
	SNATCH	60 sec.		120 sec.	L:	R:
	BEHIND THE NECK SQUAT	30 sec.		60/30/15		
	WINDMILL (LEFT AND RIGHT)	30 sec.		60/30/15		
	DOUBLE KB LONG CYCLE CLEAN	30 sec.		60/30/15		
	STAGGERED PUSH-UP (EXPLOSIVE)	30 sec.		60/30/15		
	HIGH PLANK	30 sec.		60/30/15		

heart rate	comments:
start:	
end:	
5 min. post:	

Im Athletic 6 Month Workout Plan

DATE: _____

WARM UP: CHOOSE ONE WARM FROM THE DYNAMIC FLOW DRILL LIST

Round 1

	work time	KB size	rest time	reps	
BOTTOM UP PRESS	60 sec.		90 sec.	L:	R:
SNATCH	60 sec.		90 sec.	L:	R:
DOUBLE SQUAT	30 sec.		60/30/15		
BARBELL GET-UP SIT-UP	30 sec.		60/30/15		
DOUBLE KB DEAD CLEAN	30 sec.		60/30/15		
FIGURE 8 TO A HOLD	30 sec.		60/30/15		
PUSH-UP	30 sec.		60/30/15		
PLANK	30 sec.		60/30/15		

Round 2

	work time	KB size	rest time	reps	
LONG CYCLE PRESS	60 sec.		90 sec.	L:	R:
1/2 SNATCH	60 sec.		90 sec.	L:	R:
HAND 2 HAND SUMO DEADLIFT	30 sec.		60/30/15		
SIDE BEND (LEFT AND RIGHT)	30 sec.		60/30/15		
ALTERNATING CLEAN (DIP & SWITCH)	30 sec.		60/30/15		
FIGURE 8 TO A HOLD	30 sec.		60/30/15		
CLOSE GRIP PUSH-UP (MILITARY)	30 sec.		60/30/15		

Round 3

	work time	KB size	rest time	reps	
LONG CYCLE JERK	60 sec.		90 sec.	L:	R:
1/2 SNATCH	60 sec.		90 sec.	L:	R:
BEHIND THE NECK SQUAT	30 sec.		60/30/15		
WINDMILL (LEFT AND RIGHT)	30 sec.		60/30/15		
DOUBLE KB LONG CYCLE CLEAN	30 sec.		60/30/15		
STAGGERED PUSH-UP (EXPLOSIVE)	30 sec.		60/30/15		
HIGH PLANK	30 sec.		60/30/15		

heart rate	comments:
start:	
end:	
5 min. post:	

Im Athletic 6 Month Workout Plan

DATE: _____

MONTH: 3
WEEK: 2
DAY: 2

WARM UP: CHOOSE ONE WARM FROM THE DYNAMIC FLOW DRILL LIST

		work time	KB size	rest time	reps	
Round 1	BOTTOM UP PRESS	60 sec.		90 sec.	L:	R:
	SNATCH	60 sec.		90 sec.	L:	R:
	DOUBLE SQUAT	30 sec.		60/30/15		
	BARBELL GET-UP SIT-UP	30 sec.		60/30/15		
	DOUBLE KB DEAD CLEAN	30 sec.		60/30/15		
	FIGURE 8 TO A HOLD	30 sec.		60/30/15		
	PUSH-UP	30 sec.		60/30/15		
	PLANK	30 sec.		60/30/15		

		work time	KB size	rest time	reps	
Round 2	LONG CYCLE PRESS	60 sec.		90 sec.	L:	R:
	1/2 SNATCH	60 sec.		90 sec.	L:	R:
	HAND 2 HAND SUMO DEADLIFT	30 sec.		60/30/15		
	SIDE BEND (LEFT AND RIGHT)	30 sec.		60/30/15		
	ALTERNATING CLEAN (DIP & SWITCH)	30 sec.		60/30/15		
	FIGURE 8 TO A HOLD	30 sec.		60/30/15		
	CLOSE GRIP PUSH-UP (MILITARY)	30 sec.		60/30/15		

		work time	KB size	rest time	reps	
Round 3	LONG CYCLE JERK	60 sec.		90 sec.	L:	R:
	1/2 SNATCH	60 sec.		90 sec.	L:	R:
	BEHIND THE NECK SQUAT	30 sec.		60/30/15		
	WINDMILL (LEFT AND RIGHT)	30 sec.		60/30/15		
	DOUBLE KB LONG CYCLE CLEAN	30 sec.		60/30/15		
	STAGGERED PUSH-UP (EXPLOSIVE)	30 sec.		60/30/15		
	HIGH PLANK	30 sec.		60/30/15		

heart rate	comments:
start:	
end:	
5 min. post:	

Im Athletic 6 Month Workout Plan

DATE: _____

WARM UP: CHOOSE ONE WARM FROM THE DYNAMIC FLOW DRILL LIST

		work time	KB size	rest time	reps	
Round 1	BOTTOM UP PRESS	60 sec.		90 sec.	L:	R:
	SNATCH	60 sec.		90 sec.	L:	R:
	DOUBLE SQUAT	30 sec.		60/30/15		
	BARBELL GET-UP SIT-UP	30 sec.		60/30/15		
	DOUBLE KB DEAD CLEAN	30 sec.		60/30/15		
	FIGURE 8 TO A HOLD	30 sec.		60/30/15		
	PUSH-UP	30 sec.		60/30/15		
	PLANK	30 sec.		60/30/15		

		work time	KB size	rest time	reps	
Round 2	LONG CYCLE PRESS	60 sec.		90 sec.	L:	R:
	1/2 SNATCH	60 sec.		90 sec.	L:	R:
	HAND 2 HAND SUMO DEADLIFT	30 sec.		60/30/15		
	SIDE BEND (LEFT AND RIGHT)	30 sec.		60/30/15		
	ALTERNATING CLEAN (DIP & SWITCH)	30 sec.		60/30/15		
	FIGURE 8 TO A HOLD	30 sec.		60/30/15		
	CLOSE GRIP PUSH-UP (MILITARY)	30 sec.		60/30/15		

		work time	KB size	rest time	reps	
Round 3	LONG CYCLE JERK	60 sec.		90 sec.	L:	R:
	1/2 SNATCH	60 sec.		90 sec.	L:	R:
	BEHIND THE NECK SQUAT	30 sec.		60/30/15		
	WINDMILL (LEFT AND RIGHT)	30 sec.		60/30/15		
	DOUBLE KB LONG CYCLE CLEAN	30 sec.		60/30/15		
	STAGGERED PUSH-UP (EXPLOSIVE)	30 sec.		60/30/15		
	HIGH PLANK	30 sec.		60/30/15		

heart rate	comments:
start:	
end:	
5 min. post:	

Im Athletic 6 Month Workout Plan

DATE: _____

WARM UP: CHOOSE ONE WARM FROM THE DYNAMIC FLOW DRILL LIST

		work time	KB size	rest time	reps	
Round 1	BOTTOM UP PRESS	60 sec.		90 sec.	L:	R:
	SNATCH	60 sec.		90 sec.	L:	R:
	DOUBLE SQUAT	30 sec.		60/30/15		
	BARBELL GET-UP SIT-UP	30 sec.		60/30/15		
	DOUBLE KB DEAD CLEAN	30 sec.		60/30/15		
	FIGURE 8 TO A HOLD	30 sec.		60/30/15		
	PUSH-UP	30 sec.		60/30/15		
	PLANK	30 sec.		60/30/15		

		work time	KB size	rest time	reps	
Round 2	LONG CYCLE PRESS	60 sec.		90 sec.	L:	R:
	1/2 SNATCH	60 sec.		90 sec.	L:	R:
	HAND 2 HAND SUMO DEADLIFT	30 sec.		60/30/15		
	SIDE BEND (LEFT AND RIGHT)	30 sec.		60/30/15		
	ALTERNATING CLEAN (DIP & SWITCH)	30 sec.		60/30/15		
	FIGURE 8 TO A HOLD	30 sec.		60/30/15		
	CLOSE GRIP PUSH-UP (MILITARY)	30 sec.		60/30/15		

		work time	KB size	rest time	reps	
Round 3	LONG CYCLE JERK	60 sec.		90 sec.	L:	R:
	1/2 SNATCH	60 sec.		90 sec.	L:	R:
	BEHIND THE NECK SQUAT	30 sec.		60/30/15		
	WINDMILL (LEFT AND RIGHT)	30 sec.		60/30/15		
	DOUBLE KB LONG CYCLE CLEAN	30 sec.		60/30/15		
	STAGGERED PUSH-UP (EXPLOSIVE)	30 sec.		60/30/15		
	HIGH PLANK	30 sec.		60/30/15		

heart rate	comments:
start:	
end:	
5 min. post:	

Im Athletic 6 Month Workout Plan

DATE: _____

WARM UP: CHOOSE ONE WARM FROM THE DYNAMIC FLOW DRILL LIST

		work time	KB size	rest time	reps	
Round 1	LONG CYCLE JERK	60 sec.		60 sec.	L:	R:
	1/2 SNATCH	60 sec.		60 sec.	L:	R:
	DOUBLE SQUAT	30 sec.		60/30/15		
	BARBELL GET-UP SIT-UP	30 sec.		60/30/15		
	DOUBLE KB DEAD CLEAN	30 sec.		60/30/15		
	FIGURE 8 TO A HOLD	30 sec.		60/30/15		
	PUSH-UP	30 sec.		60/30/15		
	PLANK	30 sec.		60/30/15		

		work time	KB size	rest time	reps	
Round 2	LONG CYCLE JERK	60 sec.		60 sec.	L:	R:
	1/2 SNATCH	60 sec.		60 sec.	L:	R:
	HAND 2 HAND SUMO DEADLIFT	30 sec.		60/30/15		
	SIDE BEND (LEFT AND RIGHT)	30 sec.		60/30/15		
	ALTERNATING CLEAN (DIP & SWITCH)	30 sec.		60/30/15		
	FIGURE 8 TO A HOLD	30 sec.		60/30/15		
	CLOSE GRIP PUSH-UP (MILITARY)	30 sec.		60/30/15		

		work time	KB size	rest time	reps	
Round 3	LONG CYCLE JERK	60 sec.		60 sec.	L:	R:
	1/2 SNATCH	60 sec.		60 sec.	L:	R:
	BEHIND THE NECK SQUAT	30 sec.		60/30/15		
	WINDMILL (LEFT AND RIGHT)	30 sec.		60/30/15		
	DOUBLE KB LONG CYCLE CLEAN	30 sec.		60/30/15		
	STAGGERED PUSH-UP (EXPLOSIVE)	30 sec.		60/30/15		
	HIGH PLANK	30 sec.		60/30/15		

heart rate	comments:
start:	
end:	
5 min. post:	

Im Athletic 6 Month Workout Plan

DATE: _____

WARM UP: CHOOSE ONE WARM FROM THE DYNAMIC FLOW DRILL LIST

		work time	KB size	rest time	reps	
Round 1	LONG CYCLE JERK	60 sec.		60 sec.	L:	R:
	1/2 SNATCH	60 sec.		60 sec.	L:	R:
	DOUBLE SQUAT	30 sec.		60/30/15		
	BARBELL GET-UP SIT-UP	30 sec.		60/30/15		
	DOUBLE KB DEAD CLEAN	30 sec.		60/30/15		
	FIGURE 8 TO A HOLD	30 sec.		60/30/15		
	PUSH-UP	30 sec.		60/30/15		
	PLANK	30 sec.		60/30/15		

		work time	KB size	rest time	reps	
Round 2	LONG CYCLE JERK	60 sec.		60 sec.	L:	R:
	1/2 SNATCH	60 sec.		60 sec.	L:	R:
	HAND 2 HAND SUMO DEADLIFT	30 sec.		60/30/15		
	SIDE BEND (LEFT AND RIGHT)	30 sec.		60/30/15		
	ALTERNATING CLEAN (DIP & SWITCH)	30 sec.		60/30/15		
	FIGURE 8 TO A HOLD	30 sec.		60/30/15		
	CLOSE GRIP PUSH-UP (MILITARY)	30 sec.		60/30/15		

		work time	KB size	rest time	reps	
Round 3	LONG CYCLE JERK	60 sec.		60 sec.	L:	R:
	1/2 SNATCH	60 sec.		60 sec.	L:	R:
	BEHIND THE NECK SQUAT	30 sec.		60/30/15		
	WINDMILL (LEFT AND RIGHT)	30 sec.		60/30/15		
	DOUBLE KB LONG CYCLE CLEAN	30 sec.		60/30/15		
	STAGGERED PUSH-UP (EXPLOSIVE)	30 sec.		60/30/15		
	HIGH PLANK	30 sec.		60/30/15		

heart rate	comments:
start:	
end:	
5 min. post:	

Im Athletic 6 Month Workout Plan

DATE: _____

WARM UP: CHOOSE ONE WARM FROM THE DYNAMIC FLOW DRILL LIST

		work time	KB size	rest time	reps	
Round 1	LONG CYCLE JERK	60 sec.		60 sec.	L:	R:
	1/2 SNATCH	60 sec.		60 sec.	L:	R:
	DOUBLE SQUAT	30 sec.		60/30/15		
	BARBELL GET-UP SIT-UP	30 sec.		60/30/15		
	DOUBLE KB DEAD CLEAN	30 sec.		60/30/15		
	FIGURE 8 TO A HOLD	30 sec.		60/30/15		
	PUSH-UP	30 sec.		60/30/15		
	PLANK	30 sec.		60/30/15		

		work time	KB size	rest time	reps	
Round 2	LONG CYCLE JERK	60 sec.		60 sec.	L:	R:
	1/2 SNATCH	60 sec.		60 sec.	L:	R:
	HAND 2 HAND SUMO DEADLIFT	30 sec.		60/30/15		
	SIDE BEND (LEFT AND RIGHT)	30 sec.		60/30/15		
	ALTERNATING CLEAN (DIP & SWITCH)	30 sec.		60/30/15		
	FIGURE 8 TO A HOLD	30 sec.		60/30/15		
	CLOSE GRIP PUSH-UP (MILITARY)	30 sec.		60/30/15		

		work time	KB size	rest time	reps	
Round 3	LONG CYCLE JERK	60 sec.		60 sec.	L:	R:
	1/2 SNATCH	60 sec.		60 sec.	L:	R:
	BEHIND THE NECK SQUAT	30 sec.		60/30/15		
	WINDMILL (LEFT AND RIGHT)	30 sec.		60/30/15		
	DOUBLE KB LONG CYCLE CLEAN	30 sec.		60/30/15		
	STAGGERED PUSH-UP (EXPLOSIVE)	30 sec.		60/30/15		
	HIGH PLANK	30 sec.		60/30/15		

heart rate	comments:
start:	
end:	
5 min. post:	

Im Athletic 6 Month Workout Plan

DATE: _____

WARM UP: CHOOSE ONE WARM FROM THE DYNAMIC FLOW DRILL LIST

		work time	KB size	rest time	reps	
Round 1	LONG CYCLE JERK	60 sec.		60 sec.	L:	R:
	1/2 SNATCH	60 sec.		60 sec.	L:	R:
	DOUBLE SQUAT	30 sec.		60/30/15		
	BARBELL GET-UP SIT-UP	30 sec.		60/30/15		
	DOUBLE KB DEAD CLEAN	30 sec.		60/30/15		
	FIGURE 8 TO A HOLD	30 sec.		60/30/15		
	PUSH-UP	30 sec.		60/30/15		
	PLANK	30 sec.		60/30/15		

		work time	KB size	rest time	reps	
Round 2	LONG CYCLE JERK	60 sec.		60 sec.	L:	R:
	1/2 SNATCH	60 sec.		60 sec.	L:	R:
	HAND 2 HAND SUMO DEADLIFT	30 sec.		60/30/15		
	SIDE BEND (LEFT AND RIGHT)	30 sec.		60/30/15		
	ALTERNATING CLEAN (DIP & SWITCH)	30 sec.		60/30/15		
	FIGURE 8 TO A HOLD	30 sec.		60/30/15		
	CLOSE GRIP PUSH-UP (MILITARY)	30 sec.		60/30/15		

		work time	KB size	rest time	reps	
Round 3	LONG CYCLE JERK	60 sec.		60 sec.	L:	R:
	1/2 SNATCH	60 sec.		60 sec.	L:	R:
	BEHIND THE NECK SQUAT	30 sec.		60/30/15		
	WINDMILL (LEFT AND RIGHT)	30 sec.		60/30/15		
	DOUBLE KB LONG CYCLE CLEAN	30 sec.		60/30/15		
	STAGGERED PUSH-UP (EXPLOSIVE)	30 sec.		60/30/15		
	HIGH PLANK	30 sec.		60/30/15		

heart rate	comments:
start:	
end:	
5 min. post:	

Im Athletic 6 Month Workout Plan

DATE: _____

WARM UP: CHOOSE ONE WARM FROM THE DYNAMIC FLOW DRILL LIST

		work time	KB size	rest time	reps	
Round 1	JERK	60 sec.		30 sec.	L:	R:
	SNATCH	60 sec.		30 sec.	L:	R:
	DOUBLE SQUAT	30 sec.		60/30/15		
	BARBELL GET-UP SIT-UP	30 sec.		60/30/15		
	DOUBLE KB DEAD CLEAN	30 sec.		60/30/15		
	FIGURE 8 TO A HOLD	30 sec.		60/30/15		
	PUSH-UP	30 sec.		60/30/15		
	PLANK	30 sec.		60/30/15		

		work time	KB size	rest time	reps	
Round 2	JERK	60 sec.		30 sec.	L:	R:
	SNATCH	60 sec.		30 sec.	L:	R:
	HAND 2 HAND SUMO DEADLIFT	30 sec.		60/30/15		
	SIDE BEND (LEFT AND RIGHT)	30 sec.		60/30/15		
	ALTERNATING CLEAN (DIP & SWITCH)	30 sec.		60/30/15		
	FIGURE 8 TO A HOLD	30 sec.		60/30/15		
	CLOSE GRIP PUSH-UP (MILITARY)	30 sec.		60/30/15		

		work time	KB size	rest time	reps	
Round 3	JERK	60 sec.		30 sec.	L:	R:
	SNATCH	60 sec.		30 sec.	L:	R:
	BEHIND THE NECK SQUAT	30 sec.		60/30/15		
	WINDMILL (LEFT AND RIGHT)	30 sec.		60/30/15		
	DOUBLE KB LONG CYCLE CLEAN	30 sec.		60/30/15		
	STAGGERED PUSH-UP (EXPLOSIVE)	30 sec.		60/30/15		
	HIGH PLANK	30 sec.		60/30/15		

heart rate	comments:
start:	
end:	
5 min. post:	

Im Athletic 6 Month Workout Plan

WARM UP: CHOOSE ONE WARM FROM THE DYNAMIC FLOW DRILL LIST

		work time	KB size	rest time	reps	
Round 1	JERK	60 sec.		30 sec.	L:	R:
	SNATCH	60 sec.		30 sec.	L:	R:
	DOUBLE SQUAT	30 sec.		60/30/15		
	BARBELL GET-UP SIT-UP	30 sec.		60/30/15		
	DOUBLE KB DEAD CLEAN	30 sec.		60/30/15		
	FIGURE 8 TO A HOLD	30 sec.		60/30/15		
	PUSH-UP	30 sec.		60/30/15		
	PLANK	30 sec.		60/30/15		

		work time	KB size	rest time	reps	
Round 2	JERK	60 sec.		30 sec.	L:	R:
	SNATCH	60 sec.		30 sec.	L:	R:
	HAND 2 HAND SUMO DEADLIFT	30 sec.		60/30/15		
	SIDE BEND (LEFT AND RIGHT)	30 sec.		60/30/15		
	ALTERNATING CLEAN (DIP & SWITCH)	30 sec.		60/30/15		
	FIGURE 8 TO A HOLD	30 sec.		60/30/15		
	CLOSE GRIP PUSH-UP (MILITARY)	30 sec.		60/30/15		

		work time	KB size	rest time	reps	
Round 3	JERK	60 sec.		30 sec.	L:	R:
	SNATCH	60 sec.		30 sec.	L:	R:
	BEHIND THE NECK SQUAT	30 sec.		60/30/15		
	WINDMILL (LEFT AND RIGHT)	30 sec.		60/30/15		
	DOUBLE KB LONG CYCLE CLEAN	30 sec.		60/30/15		
	STAGGERED PUSH-UP (EXPLOSIVE)	30 sec.		60/30/15		
	HIGH PLANK	30 sec.		60/30/15		

heart rate	comments:
start:	
end:	
5 min. post:	

Im Athletic 6 Month Workout Plan

DATE: _____

WARM UP: CHOOSE ONE WARM FROM THE DYNAMIC FLOW DRILL LIST

Round 1

	work time	KB size	rest time	reps	
JERK	60 sec.		30 sec.	L:	R:
SNATCH	60 sec.		30 sec.	L:	R:
DOUBLE SQUAT	30 sec.		60/30/15		
BARBELL GET-UP SIT-UP	30 sec.		60/30/15		
DOUBLE KB DEAD CLEAN	30 sec.		60/30/15		
FIGURE 8 TO A HOLD	30 sec.		60/30/15		
PUSH-UP	30 sec.		60/30/15		
PLANK	30 sec.		60/30/15		

Round 2

	work time	KB size	rest time	reps	
JERK	60 sec.		30 sec.	L:	R:
SNATCH	60 sec.		30 sec.	L:	R:
HAND 2 HAND SUMO DEADLIFT	30 sec.		60/30/15		
SIDE BEND (LEFT AND RIGHT)	30 sec.		60/30/15		
ALTERNATING CLEAN (DIP & SWITCH)	30 sec.		60/30/15		
FIGURE 8 TO A HOLD	30 sec.		60/30/15		
CLOSE GRIP PUSH-UP (MILITARY)	30 sec.		60/30/15		

Round 3

	work time	KB size	rest time	reps	
JERK	60 sec.		30 sec.	L:	R:
SNATCH	60 sec.		30 sec.	L:	R:
BEHIND THE NECK SQUAT	30 sec.		60/30/15		
WINDMILL (LEFT AND RIGHT)	30 sec.		60/30/15		
DOUBLE KB LONG CYCLE CLEAN	30 sec.		60/30/15		
STAGGERED PUSH-UP (EXPLOSIVE)	30 sec.		60/30/15		
HIGH PLANK	30 sec.		60/30/15		

heart rate	comments:
start:	
end:	
5 min. post:	

Im Athletic 6 Month Workout Plan

DATE: _____

WARM UP: CHOOSE ONE WARM FROM THE DYNAMIC FLOW DRILL LIST

		work time	KB size	rest time	reps	
Round 1	JERK	60 sec.		30 sec.	L:	R:
	SNATCH	60 sec.		30 sec.	L:	R:
	DOUBLE SQUAT	30 sec.		60/30/15		
	BARBELL GET-UP SIT-UP	30 sec.		60/30/15		
	DOUBLE KB DEAD CLEAN	30 sec.		60/30/15		
	FIGURE 8 TO A HOLD	30 sec.		60/30/15		
	PUSH-UP	30 sec.		60/30/15		
	PLANK	30 sec.		60/30/15		

		work time	KB size	rest time	reps	
Round 2	JERK	60 sec.		30 sec.	L:	R:
	SNATCH	60 sec.		30 sec.	L:	R:
	HAND 2 HAND SUMO DEADLIFT	30 sec.		60/30/15		
	SIDE BEND (LEFT AND RIGHT)	30 sec.		60/30/15		
	ALTERNATING CLEAN (DIP & SWITCH)	30 sec.		60/30/15		
	FIGURE 8 TO A HOLD	30 sec.		60/30/15		
	CLOSE GRIP PUSH-UP (MILITARY)	30 sec.		60/30/15		

		work time	KB size	rest time	reps	
Round 3	JERK	60 sec.		30 sec.	L:	R:
	SNATCH	60 sec.		30 sec.	L:	R:
	BEHIND THE NECK SQUAT	30 sec.		60/30/15		
	WINDMILL (LEFT AND RIGHT)	30 sec.		60/30/15		
	DOUBLE KB LONG CYCLE CLEAN	30 sec.		60/30/15		
	STAGGERED PUSH-UP (EXPLOSIVE)	30 sec.		60/30/15		
	HIGH PLANK	30 sec.		60/30/15		

heart rate	comments:
start:	
end:	
5 min. post:	

"Champions aren't made in the gyms. Champions are made from something they have deep inside them -- a desire, a dream, a vision."
Muhammad Ali,

Im Athletic 6 Month Workout Plan

DATE: _____

WARM UP: CHOOSE ONE WARM FROM THE DYNAMIC FLOW DRILL LIST

Round 1		work time	KB size	rest time	reps		
	JERK	90 sec.		180 sec.	L:		R:
	1/2 SNATCH	90 sec.		180 sec.	L:		R:
	DOUBLE SQUAT	30 sec.		60/30/15			
	BARBELL GET-UP SIT-UP	30 sec.		60/30/15			
	DOUBLE KB DEAD CLEAN	30 sec.		60/30/15			
	FIGURE 8 TO A HOLD	30 sec.		60/30/15			
	PUSH-UP	30 sec.		60/30/15			
	PLANK	30 sec.		60/30/15			

Round 2		work time	KB size	rest time	reps		
	PRESS	90 sec.		180 sec.	L:		R:
	1/2 SNATCH	90 sec.		180 sec.	L:		R:
	HAND 2 HAND SUMO DEADLIFT	30 sec.		60/30/15			
	SIDE BEND (LEFT AND RIGHT)	30 sec.		60/30/15			
	ALTERNATING CLEAN (DIP & SWITCH)	30 sec.		60/30/15			
	FIGURE 8 TO A HOLD	30 sec.		60/30/15			
	CLOSE GRIP PUSH-UP (MILITARY)	30 sec.		60/30/15			

Round 3		work time	KB size	rest time	reps		
	JERK	90 sec.		180 sec.	L:		R:
	SNATCH	90 sec.		180 sec.	L:		R:
	BEHIND THE NECK SQUAT	30 sec.		60/30/15			
	WINDMILL (LEFT AND RIGHT)	30 sec.		60/30/15			
	DOUBLE KB LONG CYCLE CLEAN	30 sec.		60/30/15			
	STAGGERED PUSH-UP (EXPLOSIVE)	30 sec.		60/30/15			
	HIGH PLANK	30 sec.		60/30/15			

heart rate	comments:
start:	
end:	
5 min. post:	

Im Athletic 6 Month Workout Plan

DATE: _____

WARM UP: CHOOSE ONE WARM FROM THE DYNAMIC FLOW DRILL LIST

Round 1		work time	KB size	rest time	reps	
	JERK	90 sec.		180 sec.	L:	R:
	1/2 SNATCH	90 sec.		180 sec.	L:	R:
	DOUBLE SQUAT	30 sec.		60/30/15		
	BARBELL GET-UP SIT-UP	30 sec.		60/30/15		
	DOUBLE KB DEAD CLEAN	30 sec.		60/30/15		
	FIGURE 8 TO A HOLD	30 sec.		60/30/15		
	PUSH-UP	30 sec.		60/30/15		
	PLANK	30 sec.		60/30/15		

Round 2		work time	KB size	rest time	reps	
	PRESS	90 sec.		180 sec.	L:	R:
	1/2 SNATCH	90 sec.		180 sec.	L:	R:
	HAND 2 HAND SUMO DEADLIFT	30 sec.		60/30/15		
	SIDE BEND (LEFT AND RIGHT)	30 sec.		60/30/15		
	ALTERNATING CLEAN (DIP & SWITCH)	30 sec.		60/30/15		
	FIGURE 8 TO A HOLD	30 sec.		60/30/15		
	CLOSE GRIP PUSH-UP (MILITARY)	30 sec.		60/30/15		

Round 3		work time	KB size	rest time	reps	
	JERK	90 sec.		180 sec.	L:	R:
	SNATCH	90 sec.		180 sec.	L:	R:
	BEHIND THE NECK SQUAT	30 sec.		60/30/15		
	WINDMILL (LEFT AND RIGHT)	30 sec.		60/30/15		
	DOUBLE KB LONG CYCLE CLEAN	30 sec.		60/30/15		
	STAGGERED PUSH-UP (EXPLOSIVE)	30 sec.		60/30/15		
	HIGH PLANK	30 sec.		60/30/15		

heart rate	comments:
start:	
end:	
5 min. post:	

Im Athletic 6 Month Workout Plan

DATE: _____

WARM UP: CHOOSE ONE WARM FROM THE DYNAMIC FLOW DRILL LIST

		work time	KB size	rest time	reps	
Round 1	JERK	90 sec.		180 sec.	L:	R:
	1/2 SNATCH	90 sec.		180 sec.	L:	R:
	DOUBLE SQUAT	30 sec.		60/30/15		
	BARBELL GET-UP SIT-UP	30 sec.		60/30/15		
	DOUBLE KB DEAD CLEAN	30 sec.		60/30/15		
	FIGURE 8 TO A HOLD	30 sec.		60/30/15		
	PUSH-UP	30 sec.		60/30/15		
	PLANK	30 sec.		60/30/15		

		work time	KB size	rest time	reps	
Round 2	PRESS	90 sec.		180 sec.	L:	R:
	1/2 SNATCH	90 sec.		180 sec.	L:	R:
	HAND 2 HAND SUMO DEADLIFT	30 sec.		60/30/15		
	SIDE BEND (LEFT AND RIGHT)	30 sec.		60/30/15		
	ALTERNATING CLEAN (DIP & SWITCH)	30 sec.		60/30/15		
	FIGURE 8 TO A HOLD	30 sec.		60/30/15		
	CLOSE GRIP PUSH-UP (MILITARY)	30 sec.		60/30/15		

		work time	KB size	rest time	reps	
Round 3	JERK	90 sec.		180 sec.	L:	R:
	SNATCH	90 sec.		180 sec.	L:	R:
	BEHIND THE NECK SQUAT	30 sec.		60/30/15		
	WINDMILL (LEFT AND RIGHT)	30 sec.		60/30/15		
	DOUBLE KB LONG CYCLE CLEAN	30 sec.		60/30/15		
	STAGGERED PUSH-UP (EXPLOSIVE)	30 sec.		60/30/15		
	HIGH PLANK	30 sec.		60/30/15		

heart rate	comments:
start:	
end:	
5 min. post:	

Im Athletic 6 Month Workout Plan

DATE: _____

WARM UP: CHOOSE ONE WARM FROM THE DYNAMIC FLOW DRILL LIST

		work time	KB size	rest time	reps	
Round 1	JERK	90 sec.		180 sec.	L:	R:
	1/2 SNATCH	90 sec.		180 sec.	L:	R:
	DOUBLE SQUAT	30 sec.		60/30/15		
	BARBELL GET-UP SIT-UP	30 sec.		60/30/15		
	DOUBLE KB DEAD CLEAN	30 sec.		60/30/15		
	FIGURE 8 TO A HOLD	30 sec.		60/30/15		
	PUSH-UP	30 sec.		60/30/15		
	PLANK	30 sec.		60/30/15		

		work time	KB size	rest time	reps	
Round 2	PRESS	90 sec.		180 sec.	L:	R:
	1/2 SNATCH	90 sec.		180 sec.	L:	R:
	HAND 2 HAND SUMO DEADLIFT	30 sec.		60/30/15		
	SIDE BEND (LEFT AND RIGHT)	30 sec.		60/30/15		
	ALTERNATING CLEAN (DIP & SWITCH)	30 sec.		60/30/15		
	FIGURE 8 TO A HOLD	30 sec.		60/30/15		
	CLOSE GRIP PUSH-UP (MILITARY)	30 sec.		60/30/15		

		work time	KB size	rest time	reps	
Round 3	JERK	90 sec.		180 sec.	L:	R:
	SNATCH	90 sec.		180 sec.	L:	R:
	BEHIND THE NECK SQUAT	30 sec.		60/30/15		
	WINDMILL (LEFT AND RIGHT)	30 sec.		60/30/15		
	DOUBLE KB LONG CYCLE CLEAN	30 sec.		60/30/15		
	STAGGERED PUSH-UP (EXPLOSIVE)	30 sec.		60/30/15		
	HIGH PLANK	30 sec.		60/30/15		

heart rate	comments:
start:	
end:	
5 min. post:	

Im Athletic 6 Month Workout Plan

DATE: _____

WARM UP: CHOOSE ONE WARM FROM THE DYNAMIC FLOW DRILL LIST

		work time	KB size	rest time	reps	
Round 1	BOTTOM UP PUSH PRESS	90 sec.		120 sec.	L:	R:
	1/2 SNATCH	90 sec.		120 sec.	L:	R:
	DOUBLE SQUAT	30 sec.		60/30/15		
	BARBELL GET-UP SIT-UP	30 sec.		60/30/15		
	DOUBLE KB DEAD CLEAN	30 sec.		60/30/15		
	FIGURE 8 TO A HOLD	30 sec.		60/30/15		
	PUSH-UP	30 sec.		60/30/15		
	PLANK	30 sec.		60/30/15		

		work time	KB size	rest time	reps	
Round 2	LONG CYCLE JERK	90 sec.		120 sec.	L:	R:
	SNATCH	90 sec.		120 sec.	L:	R:
	HAND 2 HAND SUMO DEADLIFT	30 sec.		60/30/15		
	SIDE BEND (LEFT AND RIGHT)	30 sec.		60/30/15		
	ALTERNATING CLEAN (DIP & SWITCH)	30 sec.		60/30/15		
	FIGURE 8 TO A HOLD	30 sec.		60/30/15		
	CLOSE GRIP PUSH-UP (MILITARY)	30 sec.		60/30/15		

		work time	KB size	rest time	reps	
Round 3	JERK	90 sec.		120 sec.	L:	R:
	SNATCH	90 sec.		120 sec.	L:	R:
	BEHIND THE NECK SQUAT	30 sec.		60/30/15		
	WINDMILL (LEFT AND RIGHT)	30 sec.		60/30/15		
	DOUBLE KB LONG CYCLE CLEAN	30 sec.		60/30/15		
	STAGGERED PUSH-UP (EXPLOSIVE)	30 sec.		60/30/15		
	HIGH PLANK	30 sec.		60/30/15		

heart rate	comments:
start:	
end:	
5 min. post:	

Im Athletic 6 Month Workout Plan

DATE: _____

WARM UP: CHOOSE ONE WARM FROM THE DYNAMIC FLOW DRILL LIST

		work time	KB size	rest time	reps	
Round 1	BOTTOM UP PUSH PRESS	90 sec.		120 sec.	L:	R:
	1/2 SNATCH	90 sec.		120 sec.	L:	R:
	DOUBLE SQUAT	30 sec.		60/30/15		
	BARBELL GET-UP SIT-UP	30 sec.		60/30/15		
	DOUBLE KB DEAD CLEAN	30 sec.		60/30/15		
	FIGURE 8 TO A HOLD	30 sec.		60/30/15		
	PUSH-UP	30 sec.		60/30/15		
	PLANK	30 sec.		60/30/15		

		work time	KB size	rest time	reps	
Round 2	LONG CYCLE JERK	90 sec.		120 sec.	L:	R:
	SNATCH	90 sec.		120 sec.	L:	R:
	HAND 2 HAND SUMO DEADLIFT	30 sec.		60/30/15		
	SIDE BEND (LEFT AND RIGHT)	30 sec.		60/30/15		
	ALTERNATING CLEAN (DIP & SWITCH)	30 sec.		60/30/15		
	FIGURE 8 TO A HOLD	30 sec.		60/30/15		
	CLOSE GRIP PUSH-UP (MILITARY)	30 sec.		60/30/15		

		work time	KB size	rest time	reps	
Round 3	JERK	90 sec.		120 sec.	L:	R:
	SNATCH	90 sec.		120 sec.	L:	R:
	BEHIND THE NECK SQUAT	30 sec.		60/30/15		
	WINDMILL (LEFT AND RIGHT)	30 sec.		60/30/15		
	DOUBLE KB LONG CYCLE CLEAN	30 sec.		60/30/15		
	STAGGERED PUSH-UP (EXPLOSIVE)	30 sec.		60/30/15		
	HIGH PLANK	30 sec.		60/30/15		

heart rate	comments:
start:	
end:	
5 min. post:	

Im Athletic 6 Month Workout Plan

DATE: _____

WARM UP: CHOOSE ONE WARM FROM THE DYNAMIC FLOW DRILL LIST

		work time	KB size	rest time	reps	
Round 1	BOTTOM UP PUSH PRESS	90 sec.		120 sec.	L:	R:
	1/2 SNATCH	90 sec.		120 sec.	L:	R:
	DOUBLE SQUAT	30 sec.		60/30/15		
	BARBELL GET-UP SIT-UP	30 sec.		60/30/15		
	DOUBLE KB DEAD CLEAN	30 sec.		60/30/15		
	FIGURE 8 TO A HOLD	30 sec.		60/30/15		
	PUSH-UP	30 sec.		60/30/15		
	PLANK	30 sec.		60/30/15		

		work time	KB size	rest time	reps	
Round 2	LONG CYCLE JERK	90 sec.		120 sec.	L:	R:
	SNATCH	90 sec.		120 sec.	L:	R:
	HAND 2 HAND SUMO DEADLIFT	30 sec.		60/30/15		
	SIDE BEND (LEFT AND RIGHT)	30 sec.		60/30/15		
	ALTERNATING CLEAN (DIP & SWITCH)	30 sec.		60/30/15		
	FIGURE 8 TO A HOLD	30 sec.		60/30/15		
	CLOSE GRIP PUSH-UP (MILITARY)	30 sec.		60/30/15		

		work time	KB size	rest time	reps	
Round 3	JERK	90 sec.		120 sec.	L:	R:
	SNATCH	90 sec.		120 sec.	L:	R:
	BEHIND THE NECK SQUAT	30 sec.		60/30/15		
	WINDMILL (LEFT AND RIGHT)	30 sec.		60/30/15		
	DOUBLE KB LONG CYCLE CLEAN	30 sec.		60/30/15		
	STAGGERED PUSH-UP (EXPLOSIVE)	30 sec.		60/30/15		
	HIGH PLANK	30 sec.		60/30/15		

heart rate	comments:
start:	
end:	
5 min. post:	

Im Athletic 6 Month Workout Plan

DATE: _____

WARM UP: CHOOSE ONE WARM FROM THE DYNAMIC FLOW DRILL LIST

		work time	KB size	rest time	reps	
Round 1	BOTTOM UP PUSH PRESS	90 sec.		120 sec.	L:	R:
	1/2 SNATCH	90 sec.		120 sec.	L:	R:
	DOUBLE SQUAT	30 sec.		60/30/15		
	BARBELL GET-UP SIT-UP	30 sec.		60/30/15		
	DOUBLE KB DEAD CLEAN	30 sec.		60/30/15		
	FIGURE 8 TO A HOLD	30 sec.		60/30/15		
	PUSH-UP	30 sec.		60/30/15		
	PLANK	30 sec.		60/30/15		

		work time	KB size	rest time	reps	
Round 2	LONG CYCLE JERK	90 sec.		120 sec.	L:	R:
	SNATCH	90 sec.		120 sec.	L:	R:
	HAND 2 HAND SUMO DEADLIFT	30 sec.		60/30/15		
	SIDE BEND (LEFT AND RIGHT)	30 sec.		60/30/15		
	ALTERNATING CLEAN (DIP & SWITCH)	30 sec.		60/30/15		
	FIGURE 8 TO A HOLD	30 sec.		60/30/15		
	CLOSE GRIP PUSH-UP (MILITARY)	30 sec.		60/30/15		

		work time	KB size	rest time	reps	
Round 3	JERK	90 sec.		120 sec.	L:	R:
	SNATCH	90 sec.		120 sec.	L:	R:
	BEHIND THE NECK SQUAT	30 sec.		60/30/15		
	WINDMILL (LEFT AND RIGHT)	30 sec.		60/30/15		
	DOUBLE KB LONG CYCLE CLEAN	30 sec.		60/30/15		
	STAGGERED PUSH-UP (EXPLOSIVE)	30 sec.		60/30/15		
	HIGH PLANK	30 sec.		60/30/15		

heart rate	comments:
start:	
end:	
5 min. post:	

Im Athletic 6 Month Workout Plan

DATE: _____

WARM UP: CHOOSE ONE WARM FROM THE DYNAMIC FLOW DRILL LIST

Round 1

	work time	KB size	rest time	reps	
LONG CYCLE PUSH PRESS	90 sec.		90 sec.	L:	R:
1/2 SNATCH	90 sec.		90 sec.	L:	R:
DOUBLE SQUAT	30 sec.		60/30/15		
BARBELL GET-UP SIT-UP	30 sec.		60/30/15		
DOUBLE KB DEAD CLEAN	30 sec.		60/30/15		
FIGURE 8 TO A HOLD	30 sec.		60/30/15		
PUSH-UP	30 sec.		60/30/15		
PLANK	30 sec.		60/30/15		

Round 2

	work time	KB size	rest time	reps	
BOTTOM UP JERK	90 sec.		90 sec.	L:	R:
SNATCH	90 sec.		90 sec.	L:	R:
HAND 2 HAND SUMO DEADLIFT	30 sec.		60/30/15		
SIDE BEND (LEFT AND RIGHT)	30 sec.		60/30/15		
ALTERNATING CLEAN (DIP & SWITCH)	30 sec.		60/30/15		
FIGURE 8 TO A HOLD	30 sec.		60/30/15		
CLOSE GRIP PUSH-UP (MILITARY)	30 sec.		60/30/15		

Round 3

	work time	KB size	rest time	reps	
JERK	90 sec.		90 sec.	L:	R:
SNATCH	90 sec.		90 sec.	L:	R:
BEHIND THE NECK SQUAT	30 sec.		60/30/15		
WINDMILL (LEFT AND RIGHT)	30 sec.		60/30/15		
DOUBLE KB LONG CYCLE CLEAN	30 sec.		60/30/15		
STAGGERED PUSH-UP (EXPLOSIVE)	30 sec.		60/30/15		
HIGH PLANK	30 sec.		60/30/15		

heart rate	comments:
start:	
end:	
5 min. post:	

Im Athletic 6 Month Workout Plan

DATE: _____

WARM UP: CHOOSE ONE WARM FROM THE DYNAMIC FLOW DRILL LIST

		work time	KB size	rest time	reps	
Round 1	LONG CYCLE PUSH PRESS	90 sec.		90 sec.	L:	R:
	1/2 SNATCH	90 sec.		90 sec.	L:	R:
	DOUBLE SQUAT	30 sec.		60/30/15		
	BARBELL GET-UP SIT-UP	30 sec.		60/30/15		
	DOUBLE KB DEAD CLEAN	30 sec.		60/30/15		
	FIGURE 8 TO A HOLD	30 sec.		60/30/15		
	PUSH-UP	30 sec.		60/30/15		
	PLANK	30 sec.		60/30/15		

		work time	KB size	rest time	reps	
Round 2	BOTTOM UP JERK	90 sec.		90 sec.	L:	R:
	SNATCH	90 sec.		90 sec.	L:	R:
	HAND 2 HAND SUMO DEADLIFT	30 sec.		60/30/15		
	SIDE BEND (LEFT AND RIGHT)	30 sec.		60/30/15		
	ALTERNATING CLEAN (DIP & SWITCH)	30 sec.		60/30/15		
	FIGURE 8 TO A HOLD	30 sec.		60/30/15		
	CLOSE GRIP PUSH-UP (MILITARY)	30 sec.		60/30/15		

		work time	KB size	rest time	reps	
Round 3	JERK	90 sec.		90 sec.	L:	R:
	SNATCH	90 sec.		90 sec.	L:	R:
	BEHIND THE NECK SQUAT	30 sec.		60/30/15		
	WINDMILL (LEFT AND RIGHT)	30 sec.		60/30/15		
	DOUBLE KB LONG CYCLE CLEAN	30 sec.		60/30/15		
	STAGGERED PUSH-UP (EXPLOSIVE)	30 sec.		60/30/15		
	HIGH PLANK	30 sec.		60/30/15		

heart rate	comments:
start:	
end:	
5 min. post:	

Im Athletic 6 Month Workout Plan

DATE: _____

WARM UP: CHOOSE ONE WARM FROM THE DYNAMIC FLOW DRILL LIST

Round 1		work time	KB size	rest time	reps	
	LONG CYCLE PUSH PRESS	90 sec.		90 sec.	L:	R:
	1/2 SNATCH	90 sec.		90 sec.	L:	R:
	DOUBLE SQUAT	30 sec.		60/30/15		
	BARBELL GET-UP SIT-UP	30 sec.		60/30/15		
	DOUBLE KB DEAD CLEAN	30 sec.		60/30/15		
	FIGURE 8 TO A HOLD	30 sec.		60/30/15		
	PUSH-UP	30 sec.		60/30/15		
	PLANK	30 sec.		60/30/15		

Round 2		work time	KB size	rest time	reps	
	BOTTOM UP JERK	90 sec.		90 sec.	L:	R:
	SNATCH	90 sec.		90 sec.	L:	R:
	HAND 2 HAND SUMO DEADLIFT	30 sec.		60/30/15		
	SIDE BEND (LEFT AND RIGHT)	30 sec.		60/30/15		
	ALTERNATING CLEAN (DIP & SWITCH)	30 sec.		60/30/15		
	FIGURE 8 TO A HOLD	30 sec.		60/30/15		
	CLOSE GRIP PUSH-UP (MILITARY)	30 sec.		60/30/15		

Round 3		work time	KB size	rest time	reps	
	JERK	90 sec.		90 sec.	L:	R:
	SNATCH	90 sec.		90 sec.	L:	R:
	BEHIND THE NECK SQUAT	30 sec.		60/30/15		
	WINDMILL (LEFT AND RIGHT)	30 sec.		60/30/15		
	DOUBLE KB LONG CYCLE CLEAN	30 sec.		60/30/15		
	STAGGERED PUSH-UP (EXPLOSIVE)	30 sec.		60/30/15		
	HIGH PLANK	30 sec.		60/30/15		

heart rate	comments:
start:	
end:	
5 min. post:	

Im Athletic 6 Month Workout Plan

DATE: _____

WARM UP: CHOOSE ONE WARM FROM THE DYNAMIC FLOW DRILL LIST

Round 1		work time	KB size	rest time	reps	
	LONG CYCLE PUSH PRESS	90 sec.		90 sec.	L:	R:
	1/2 SNATCH	90 sec.		90 sec.	L:	R:
	DOUBLE SQUAT	30 sec.		60/30/15		
	BARBELL GET-UP SIT-UP	30 sec.		60/30/15		
	DOUBLE KB DEAD CLEAN	30 sec.		60/30/15		
	FIGURE 8 TO A HOLD	30 sec.		60/30/15		
	PUSH-UP	30 sec.		60/30/15		
	PLANK	30 sec.		60/30/15		

Round 2		work time	KB size	rest time	reps	
	BOTTOM UP JERK	90 sec.		90 sec.	L:	R:
	SNATCH	90 sec.		90 sec.	L:	R:
	HAND 2 HAND SUMO DEADLIFT	30 sec.		60/30/15		
	SIDE BEND (LEFT AND RIGHT)	30 sec.		60/30/15		
	ALTERNATING CLEAN (DIP & SWITCH)	30 sec.		60/30/15		
	FIGURE 8 TO A HOLD	30 sec.		60/30/15		
	CLOSE GRIP PUSH-UP (MILITARY)	30 sec.		60/30/15		

Round 3		work time	KB size	rest time	reps	
	JERK	90 sec.		90 sec.	L:	R:
	SNATCH	90 sec.		90 sec.	L:	R:
	BEHIND THE NECK SQUAT	30 sec.		60/30/15		
	WINDMILL (LEFT AND RIGHT)	30 sec.		60/30/15		
	DOUBLE KB LONG CYCLE CLEAN	30 sec.		60/30/15		
	STAGGERED PUSH-UP (EXPLOSIVE)	30 sec.		60/30/15		
	HIGH PLANK	30 sec.		60/30/15		

heart rate	comments:
start:	
end:	
5 min. post:	

Im Athletic 6 Month Workout Plan

DATE: _____

MONTH: 4
WEEK: 4
DAY: 1

WARM UP: CHOOSE ONE WARM FROM THE DYNAMIC FLOW DRILL LIST

Round 1

	work time	KB size	rest time	reps	
LONG CYCLE PRESS	90 sec.		45 sec.	L:	R:
SNATCH	90 sec.		45 sec.	L:	R:
DOUBLE SQUAT	30 sec.		60/30/15		
BARBELL GET-UP SIT-UP	30 sec.		60/30/15		
DOUBLE KB DEAD CLEAN	30 sec.		60/30/15		
FIGURE 8 TO A HOLD	30 sec.		60/30/15		
PUSH-UP	30 sec.		60/30/15		
PLANK	30 sec.		60/30/15		

Round 2

	work time	KB size	rest time	reps	
LONG CYCLE JERK	90 sec.		45 sec.	L:	R:
SNATCH	90 sec.		45 sec.	L:	R:
HAND 2 HAND SUMO DEADLIFT	30 sec.		60/30/15		
SIDE BEND (LEFT AND RIGHT)	30 sec.		60/30/15		
ALTERNATING CLEAN (DIP & SWITCH)	30 sec.		60/30/15		
FIGURE 8 TO A HOLD	30 sec.		60/30/15		
CLOSE GRIP PUSH-UP (MILITARY)	30 sec.		60/30/15		

Round 3

	work time	KB size	rest time	reps	
PUSH PRESS	90 sec.		45 sec.	L:	R:
1/2 SNATCH	90 sec.		45 sec.	L:	R:
BEHIND THE NECK SQUAT	30 sec.		60/30/15		
WINDMILL (LEFT AND RIGHT)	30 sec.		60/30/15		
DOUBLE KB LONG CYCLE CLEAN	30 sec.		60/30/15		
STAGGERED PUSH-UP (EXPLOSIVE)	30 sec.		60/30/15		
HIGH PLANK	30 sec.		60/30/15		

heart rate	comments:
start:	
end:	
5 min. post:	

Im Athletic 6 Month Workout Plan

DATE: _____

WARM UP: CHOOSE ONE WARM FROM THE DYNAMIC FLOW DRILL LIST

		work time	KB size	rest time	reps	
Round 1	LONG CYCLE PRESS	90 sec.		45 sec.	L:	R:
	SNATCH	90 sec.		45 sec.	L:	R:
	DOUBLE SQUAT	30 sec.		60/30/15		
	BARBELL GET-UP SIT-UP	30 sec.		60/30/15		
	DOUBLE KB DEAD CLEAN	30 sec.		60/30/15		
	FIGURE 8 TO A HOLD	30 sec.		60/30/15		
	PUSH-UP	30 sec.		60/30/15		
	PLANK	30 sec.		60/30/15		

		work time	KB size	rest time	reps	
Round 2	LONG CYCLE JERK	90 sec.		45 sec.	L:	R:
	SNATCH	90 sec.		45 sec.	L:	R:
	HAND 2 HAND SUMO DEADLIFT	30 sec.		60/30/15		
	SIDE BEND (LEFT AND RIGHT)	30 sec.		60/30/15		
	ALTERNATING CLEAN (DIP & SWITCH)	30 sec.		60/30/15		
	FIGURE 8 TO A HOLD	30 sec.		60/30/15		
	CLOSE GRIP PUSH-UP (MILITARY)	30 sec.		60/30/15		

		work time	KB size	rest time	reps	
Round 3	PUSH PRESS	90 sec.		45 sec.	L:	R:
	1/2 SNATCH	90 sec.		45 sec.	L:	R:
	BEHIND THE NECK SQUAT	30 sec.		60/30/15		
	WINDMILL (LEFT AND RIGHT)	30 sec.		60/30/15		
	DOUBLE KB LONG CYCLE CLEAN	30 sec.		60/30/15		
	STAGGERED PUSH-UP (EXPLOSIVE)	30 sec.		60/30/15		
	HIGH PLANK	30 sec.		60/30/15		

heart rate	comments:
start:	
end:	
5 min. post:	

Im Athletic 6 Month Workout Plan

DATE: _____

WARM UP: CHOOSE ONE WARM FROM THE DYNAMIC FLOW DRILL LIST

Round 1

	work time	KB size	rest time	reps	
LONG CYCLE PRESS	90 sec.		45 sec.	L:	R:
SNATCH	90 sec.		45 sec.	L:	R:
DOUBLE SQUAT	30 sec.		60/30/15		
BARBELL GET-UP SIT-UP	30 sec.		60/30/15		
DOUBLE KB DEAD CLEAN	30 sec.		60/30/15		
FIGURE 8 TO A HOLD	30 sec.		60/30/15		
PUSH-UP	30 sec.		60/30/15		
PLANK	30 sec.		60/30/15		

Round 2

	work time	KB size	rest time	reps	
LONG CYCLE JERK	90 sec.		45 sec.	L:	R:
SNATCH	90 sec.		45 sec.	L:	R:
HAND 2 HAND SUMO DEADLIFT	30 sec.		60/30/15		
SIDE BEND (LEFT AND RIGHT)	30 sec.		60/30/15		
ALTERNATING CLEAN (DIP & SWITCH)	30 sec.		60/30/15		
FIGURE 8 TO A HOLD	30 sec.		60/30/15		
CLOSE GRIP PUSH-UP (MILITARY)	30 sec.		60/30/15		

Round 3

	work time	KB size	rest time	reps	
PUSH PRESS	90 sec.		45 sec.	L:	R:
1/2 SNATCH	90 sec.		45 sec.	L:	R:
BEHIND THE NECK SQUAT	30 sec.		60/30/15		
WINDMILL (LEFT AND RIGHT)	30 sec.		60/30/15		
DOUBLE KB LONG CYCLE CLEAN	30 sec.		60/30/15		
STAGGERED PUSH-UP (EXPLOSIVE)	30 sec.		60/30/15		
HIGH PLANK	30 sec.		60/30/15		

heart rate	comments:
start:	
end:	
5 min. post:	

Im Athletic 6 Month Workout Plan

DATE: _____

WARM UP: CHOOSE ONE WARM FROM THE DYNAMIC FLOW DRILL LIST

Round 1

	work time	KB size	rest time	reps	
LONG CYCLE PRESS	90 sec.		45 sec.	L:	R:
SNATCH	90 sec.		45 sec.	L:	R:
DOUBLE SQUAT	30 sec.		60/30/15		
BARBELL GET-UP SIT-UP	30 sec.		60/30/15		
DOUBLE KB DEAD CLEAN	30 sec.		60/30/15		
FIGURE 8 TO A HOLD	30 sec.		60/30/15		
PUSH-UP	30 sec.		60/30/15		
PLANK	30 sec.		60/30/15		

Round 2

	work time	KB size	rest time	reps	
LONG CYCLE JERK	90 sec.		45 sec.	L:	R:
SNATCH	90 sec.		45 sec.	L:	R:
HAND 2 HAND SUMO DEADLIFT	30 sec.		60/30/15		
SIDE BEND (LEFT AND RIGHT)	30 sec.		60/30/15		
ALTERNATING CLEAN (DIP & SWITCH)	30 sec.		60/30/15		
FIGURE 8 TO A HOLD	30 sec.		60/30/15		
CLOSE GRIP PUSH-UP (MILITARY)	30 sec.		60/30/15		

Round 3

	work time	KB size	rest time	reps	
PUSH PRESS	90 sec.		45 sec.	L:	R:
1/2 SNATCH	90 sec.		45 sec.	L:	R:
BEHIND THE NECK SQUAT	30 sec.		60/30/15		
WINDMILL (LEFT AND RIGHT)	30 sec.		60/30/15		
DOUBLE KB LONG CYCLE CLEAN	30 sec.		60/30/15		
STAGGERED PUSH-UP (EXPLOSIVE)	30 sec.		60/30/15		
HIGH PLANK	30 sec.		60/30/15		

heart rate	comments:
start:	
end:	
5 min. post:	

You've finished month 4!

Benefit No. 2 to Kettlebell training:

Displaced Center of Gravity: The kettlebell's center of gravity is 6-8 inches below the center of your hand. Barbells and dumbbells center the weight with your hand. This center displacement, combined with the type of routines, incorporates more core strength into your workout. Kettlebells can do what dumbbells can do, better in fact, but not vice-versa.

Im Athletic 6 Month Workout Plan

DATE: _____

MONTH: 5
WEEK: 1
DAY: 1

WARM UP: CHOOSE ONE WARM FROM THE DYNAMIC FLOW DRILL LIST

		work time	KB size	rest time	reps	
Round 1	JERK	120 sec.		120 sec.	L:	R:
	SNATCH	120 sec.		120 sec.	L:	R:
	DOUBLE SQUAT	30 sec.		60/30/15		
	BARBELL GET-UP SIT-UP	30 sec.		60/30/15		
	DOUBLE KB DEAD CLEAN	30 sec.		60/30/15		
	FIGURE 8 TO A HOLD	30 sec.		60/30/15		
	PUSH-UP	30 sec.		60/30/15		
	PLANK	30 sec.		60/30/15		

		work time	KB size	rest time	reps	
Round 2	LONG CYCLE JERK	120 sec.		120 sec.	L:	R:
	1/2 SNATCH	120 sec.		120 sec.	L:	R:
	HAND 2 HAND SUMO DEADLIFT	30 sec.		60/30/15		
	SIDE BEND (LEFT AND RIGHT)	30 sec.		60/30/15		
	ALTERNATING CLEAN (DIP & SWITCH)	30 sec.		60/30/15		
	FIGURE 8 TO A HOLD	30 sec.		60/30/15		
	CLOSE GRIP PUSH-UP (MILITARY)	30 sec.		60/30/15		

		work time	KB size	rest time	reps	
Round 3	LONG CYCLE PRESS	120 sec.		120 sec.	L:	R:
	1/2 SNATCH	120 sec.		120 sec.	L:	R:
	BEHIND THE NECK SQUAT	30 sec.		60/30/15		
	WINDMILL (LEFT AND RIGHT)	30 sec.		60/30/15		
	DOUBLE KB LONG CYCLE CLEAN	30 sec.		60/30/15		
	STAGGERED PUSH-UP (EXPLOSIVE)	30 sec.		60/30/15		
	HIGH PLANK	30 sec.		60/30/15		

heart rate	comments:
start:	
end:	
5 min. post:	

Im Athletic 6 Month Workout Plan

DATE: _____

WARM UP: CHOOSE ONE WARM FROM THE DYNAMIC FLOW DRILL LIST

Round 1		work time	KB size	rest time	reps	
	JERK	120 sec.		120 sec.	L:	R:
	SNATCH	120 sec.		120 sec.	L:	R:
	DOUBLE SQUAT	30 sec.		60/30/15		
	BARBELL GET-UP SIT-UP	30 sec.		60/30/15		
	DOUBLE KB DEAD CLEAN	30 sec.		60/30/15		
	FIGURE 8 TO A HOLD	30 sec.		60/30/15		
	PUSH-UP	30 sec.		60/30/15		
	PLANK	30 sec.		60/30/15		

Round 2		work time	KB size	rest time	reps	
	LONG CYCLE JERK	120 sec.		120 sec.	L:	R:
	1/2 SNATCH	120 sec.		120 sec.	L:	R:
	HAND 2 HAND SUMO DEADLIFT	30 sec.		60/30/15		
	SIDE BEND (LEFT AND RIGHT)	30 sec.		60/30/15		
	ALTERNATING CLEAN (DIP & SWITCH)	30 sec.		60/30/15		
	FIGURE 8 TO A HOLD	30 sec.		60/30/15		
	CLOSE GRIP PUSH-UP (MILITARY)	30 sec.		60/30/15		

Round 3		work time	KB size	rest time	reps	
	LONG CYCLE PRESS	120 sec.		120 sec.	L:	R:
	1/2 SNATCH	120 sec.		120 sec.	L:	R:
	BEHIND THE NECK SQUAT	30 sec.		60/30/15		
	WINDMILL (LEFT AND RIGHT)	30 sec.		60/30/15		
	DOUBLE KB LONG CYCLE CLEAN	30 sec.		60/30/15		
	STAGGERED PUSH-UP (EXPLOSIVE)	30 sec.		60/30/15		
	HIGH PLANK	30 sec.		60/30/15		

heart rate	comments:
start:	
end:	
5 min. post:	

Im Athletic 6 Month Workout Plan

DATE: _____

MONTH: 5
WEEK: 1
DAY: 3

WARM UP: CHOOSE ONE WARM FROM THE DYNAMIC FLOW DRILL LIST

Round 1		work time	KB size	rest time	reps	
	JERK	120 sec.		120 sec.	L:	R:
	SNATCH	120 sec.		120 sec.	L:	R:
	DOUBLE SQUAT	30 sec.		60/30/15		
	BARBELL GET-UP SIT-UP	30 sec.		60/30/15		
	DOUBLE KB DEAD CLEAN	30 sec.		60/30/15		
	FIGURE 8 TO A HOLD	30 sec.		60/30/15		
	PUSH-UP	30 sec.		60/30/15		
	PLANK	30 sec.		60/30/15		

Round 2		work time	KB size	rest time	reps	
	LONG CYCLE JERK	120 sec.		120 sec.	L:	R:
	1/2 SNATCH	120 sec.		120 sec.	L:	R:
	HAND 2 HAND SUMO DEADLIFT	30 sec.		60/30/15		
	SIDE BEND (LEFT AND RIGHT)	30 sec.		60/30/15		
	ALTERNATING CLEAN (DIP & SWITCH)	30 sec.		60/30/15		
	FIGURE 8 TO A HOLD	30 sec.		60/30/15		
	CLOSE GRIP PUSH-UP (MILITARY)	30 sec.		60/30/15		

Round 3		work time	KB size	rest time	reps	
	LONG CYCLE PRESS	120 sec.		120 sec.	L:	R:
	1/2 SNATCH	120 sec.		120 sec.	L:	R:
	BEHIND THE NECK SQUAT	30 sec.		60/30/15		
	WINDMILL (LEFT AND RIGHT)	30 sec.		60/30/15		
	DOUBLE KB LONG CYCLE CLEAN	30 sec.		60/30/15		
	STAGGERED PUSH-UP (EXPLOSIVE)	30 sec.		60/30/15		
	HIGH PLANK	30 sec.		60/30/15		

heart rate	comments:
start:	
end:	
5 min. post:	

Im Athletic 6 Month Workout Plan

DATE: _____

WARM UP: CHOOSE ONE WARM FROM THE DYNAMIC FLOW DRILL LIST

Round 1

	work time	KB size	rest time	reps	
JERK	120 sec.		120 sec.	L:	R:
SNATCH	120 sec.		120 sec.	L:	R:
DOUBLE SQUAT	30 sec.		60/30/15		
BARBELL GET-UP SIT-UP	30 sec.		60/30/15		
DOUBLE KB DEAD CLEAN	30 sec.		60/30/15		
FIGURE 8 TO A HOLD	30 sec.		60/30/15		
PUSH-UP	30 sec.		60/30/15		
PLANK	30 sec.		60/30/15		

Round 2

	work time	KB size	rest time	reps	
LONG CYCLE JERK	120 sec.		120 sec.	L:	R:
1/2 SNATCH	120 sec.		120 sec.	L:	R:
HAND 2 HAND SUMO DEADLIFT	30 sec.		60/30/15		
SIDE BEND (LEFT AND RIGHT)	30 sec.		60/30/15		
ALTERNATING CLEAN (DIP & SWITCH)	30 sec.		60/30/15		
FIGURE 8 TO A HOLD	30 sec.		60/30/15		
CLOSE GRIP PUSH-UP (MILITARY)	30 sec.		60/30/15		

Round 3

	work time	KB size	rest time	reps	
LONG CYCLE PRESS	120 sec.		120 sec.	L:	R:
1/2 SNATCH	120 sec.		120 sec.	L:	R:
BEHIND THE NECK SQUAT	30 sec.		60/30/15		
WINDMILL (LEFT AND RIGHT)	30 sec.		60/30/15		
DOUBLE KB LONG CYCLE CLEAN	30 sec.		60/30/15		
STAGGERED PUSH-UP (EXPLOSIVE)	30 sec.		60/30/15		
HIGH PLANK	30 sec.		60/30/15		

heart rate	comments:
start:	
end:	
5 min. post:	

Im Athletic 6 Month Workout Plan

WARM UP: CHOOSE ONE WARM FROM THE DYNAMIC FLOW DRILL LIST

		work time	KB size	rest time	reps	
Round 1	JERK	120 sec.		90 sec.	L:	R:
	SNATCH	120 sec.		90 sec.	L:	R:
	DOUBLE SQUAT	30 sec.		60/30/15		
	BARBELL GET-UP SIT-UP	30 sec.		60/30/15		
	DOUBLE KB DEAD CLEAN	30 sec.		60/30/15		
	FIGURE 8 TO A HOLD	30 sec.		60/30/15		
	PUSH-UP	30 sec.		60/30/15		
	PLANK	30 sec.		60/30/15		

		work time	KB size	rest time	reps	
Round 2	JERK	120 sec.		90 sec.	L:	R:
	1/2 SNATCH	120 sec.		90 sec.	L:	R:
	HAND 2 HAND SUMO DEADLIFT	30 sec.		60/30/15		
	SIDE BEND (LEFT AND RIGHT)	30 sec.		60/30/15		
	ALTERNATING CLEAN (DIP & SWITCH)	30 sec.		60/30/15		
	FIGURE 8 TO A HOLD	30 sec.		60/30/15		
	CLOSE GRIP PUSH-UP (MILITARY)	30 sec.		60/30/15		

		work time	KB size	rest time	reps	
Round 3	LONG CYCLE JERK	120 sec.		90 sec.	L:	R:
	SNATCH	120 sec.		90 sec.	L:	R:
	BEHIND THE NECK SQUAT	30 sec.		60/30/15		
	WINDMILL (LEFT AND RIGHT)	30 sec.		60/30/15		
	DOUBLE KB LONG CYCLE CLEAN	30 sec.		60/30/15		
	STAGGERED PUSH-UP (EXPLOSIVE)	30 sec.		60/30/15		
	HIGH PLANK	30 sec.		60/30/15		

heart rate	comments:
start:	
end:	
5 min. post:	

Im Athletic 6 Month Workout Plan

DATE: _____

WARM UP: CHOOSE ONE WARM FROM THE DYNAMIC FLOW DRILL LIST

		work time	KB size	rest time	reps	
Round 1	JERK	120 sec.		90 sec.	L:	R:
	SNATCH	120 sec.		90 sec.	L:	R:
	DOUBLE SQUAT	30 sec.		60/30/15		
	BARBELL GET-UP SIT-UP	30 sec.		60/30/15		
	DOUBLE KB DEAD CLEAN	30 sec.		60/30/15		
	FIGURE 8 TO A HOLD	30 sec.		60/30/15		
	PUSH-UP	30 sec.		60/30/15		
	PLANK	30 sec.		60/30/15		

		work time	KB size	rest time	reps	
Round 2	JERK	120 sec.		90 sec.	L:	R:
	1/2 SNATCH	120 sec.		90 sec.	L:	R:
	HAND 2 HAND SUMO DEADLIFT	30 sec.		60/30/15		
	SIDE BEND (LEFT AND RIGHT)	30 sec.		60/30/15		
	ALTERNATING CLEAN (DIP & SWITCH)	30 sec.		60/30/15		
	FIGURE 8 TO A HOLD	30 sec.		60/30/15		
	CLOSE GRIP PUSH-UP (MILITARY)	30 sec.		60/30/15		

		work time	KB size	rest time	reps	
Round 3	LONG CYCLE JERK	120 sec.		90 sec.	L:	R:
	SNATCH	120 sec.		90 sec.	L:	R:
	BEHIND THE NECK SQUAT	30 sec.		60/30/15		
	WINDMILL (LEFT AND RIGHT)	30 sec.		60/30/15		
	DOUBLE KB LONG CYCLE CLEAN	30 sec.		60/30/15		
	STAGGERED PUSH-UP (EXPLOSIVE)	30 sec.		60/30/15		
	HIGH PLANK	30 sec.		60/30/15		

heart rate	comments:
start:	
end:	
5 min. post:	

Im Athletic 6 Month Workout Plan

DATE: _____

WARM UP: CHOOSE ONE WARM FROM THE DYNAMIC FLOW DRILL LIST

		work time	KB size	rest time	reps	
Round 1	JERK	120 sec.		90 sec.	L:	R:
	SNATCH	120 sec.		90 sec.	L:	R:
	DOUBLE SQUAT	30 sec.		60/30/15		
	BARBELL GET-UP SIT-UP	30 sec.		60/30/15		
	DOUBLE KB DEAD CLEAN	30 sec.		60/30/15		
	FIGURE 8 TO A HOLD	30 sec.		60/30/15		
	PUSH-UP	30 sec.		60/30/15		
	PLANK	30 sec.		60/30/15		

		work time	KB size	rest time	reps	
Round 2	JERK	120 sec.		90 sec.	L:	R:
	1/2 SNATCH	120 sec.		90 sec.	L:	R:
	HAND 2 HAND SUMO DEADLIFT	30 sec.		60/30/15		
	SIDE BEND (LEFT AND RIGHT)	30 sec.		60/30/15		
	ALTERNATING CLEAN (DIP & SWITCH)	30 sec.		60/30/15		
	FIGURE 8 TO A HOLD	30 sec.		60/30/15		
	CLOSE GRIP PUSH-UP (MILITARY)	30 sec.		60/30/15		

		work time	KB size	rest time	reps	
Round 3	LONG CYCLE JERK	120 sec.		90 sec.	L:	R:
	SNATCH	120 sec.		90 sec.	L:	R:
	BEHIND THE NECK SQUAT	30 sec.		60/30/15		
	WINDMILL (LEFT AND RIGHT)	30 sec.		60/30/15		
	DOUBLE KB LONG CYCLE CLEAN	30 sec.		60/30/15		
	STAGGERED PUSH-UP (EXPLOSIVE)	30 sec.		60/30/15		
	HIGH PLANK	30 sec.		60/30/15		

heart rate	comments:
start:	
end:	
5 min. post:	

Im Athletic 6 Month Workout Plan

DATE: _____

WARM UP: CHOOSE ONE WARM FROM THE DYNAMIC FLOW DRILL LIST

		work time	KB size	rest time	reps	
Round 1	JERK	120 sec.		90 sec.	L:	R:
	SNATCH	120 sec.		90 sec.	L:	R:
	DOUBLE SQUAT	30 sec.		60/30/15		
	BARBELL GET-UP SIT-UP	30 sec.		60/30/15		
	DOUBLE KB DEAD CLEAN	30 sec.		60/30/15		
	FIGURE 8 TO A HOLD	30 sec.		60/30/15		
	PUSH-UP	30 sec.		60/30/15		
	PLANK	30 sec.		60/30/15		

		work time	KB size	rest time	reps	
Round 2	JERK	120 sec.		90 sec.	L:	R:
	1/2 SNATCH	120 sec.		90 sec.	L:	R:
	HAND 2 HAND SUMO DEADLIFT	30 sec.		60/30/15		
	SIDE BEND (LEFT AND RIGHT)	30 sec.		60/30/15		
	ALTERNATING CLEAN (DIP & SWITCH)	30 sec.		60/30/15		
	FIGURE 8 TO A HOLD	30 sec.		60/30/15		
	CLOSE GRIP PUSH-UP (MILITARY)	30 sec.		60/30/15		

		work time	KB size	rest time	reps	
Round 3	LONG CYCLE JERK	120 sec.		90 sec.	L:	R:
	SNATCH	120 sec.		90 sec.	L:	R:
	BEHIND THE NECK SQUAT	30 sec.		60/30/15		
	WINDMILL (LEFT AND RIGHT)	30 sec.		60/30/15		
	DOUBLE KB LONG CYCLE CLEAN	30 sec.		60/30/15		
	STAGGERED PUSH-UP (EXPLOSIVE)	30 sec.		60/30/15		
	HIGH PLANK	30 sec.		60/30/15		

heart rate	comments:
start:	
end:	
5 min. post:	

Im Athletic 6 Month Workout Plan

DATE: _____

WARM UP: CHOOSE ONE WARM FROM THE DYNAMIC FLOW DRILL LIST

		work time	KB size	rest time	reps	
Round 1	BOTTOM UP JERK	120 sec.		60 sec.	L:	R:
	SNATCH	120 sec.		60 sec.	L:	R:
	DOUBLE SQUAT	30 sec.		60/30/15		
	BARBELL GET-UP SIT-UP	30 sec.		60/30/15		
	DOUBLE KB DEAD CLEAN	30 sec.		60/30/15		
	FIGURE 8 TO A HOLD	30 sec.		60/30/15		
	PUSH-UP	30 sec.		60/30/15		
	PLANK	30 sec.		60/30/15		

		work time	KB size	rest time	reps	
Round 2	LONG CYCLE JERK	120 sec.		60 sec.	L:	R:
	1/2 SNATCH	120 sec.		60 sec.	L:	R:
	HAND 2 HAND SUMO DEADLIFT	30 sec.		60/30/15		
	SIDE BEND (LEFT AND RIGHT)	30 sec.		60/30/15		
	ALTERNATING CLEAN (DIP & SWITCH)	30 sec.		60/30/15		
	FIGURE 8 TO A HOLD	30 sec.		60/30/15		
	CLOSE GRIP PUSH-UP (MILITARY)	30 sec.		60/30/15		

		work time	KB size	rest time	reps	
Round 3	PRESS	120 sec.		60 sec.	L:	R:
	SNATCH	120 sec.		60 sec.	L:	R:
	BEHIND THE NECK SQUAT	30 sec.		60/30/15		
	WINDMILL (LEFT AND RIGHT)	30 sec.		60/30/15		
	DOUBLE KB LONG CYCLE CLEAN	30 sec.		60/30/15		
	STAGGERED PUSH-UP (EXPLOSIVE)	30 sec.		60/30/15		
	HIGH PLANK	30 sec.		60/30/15		

heart rate	comments:
start:	
end:	
5 min. post:	

Im Athletic 6 Month Workout Plan

DATE: _____

WARM UP: CHOOSE ONE WARM FROM THE DYNAMIC FLOW DRILL LIST

		work time	KB size	rest time	reps	
Round 1	BOTTOM UP JERK	120 sec.		60 sec.	L:	R:
	SNATCH	120 sec.		60 sec.	L:	R:
	DOUBLE SQUAT	30 sec.		60/30/15		
	BARBELL GET-UP SIT-UP	30 sec.		60/30/15		
	DOUBLE KB DEAD CLEAN	30 sec.		60/30/15		
	FIGURE 8 TO A HOLD	30 sec.		60/30/15		
	PUSH-UP	30 sec.		60/30/15		
	PLANK	30 sec.		60/30/15		

		work time	KB size	rest time	reps	
Round 2	LONG CYCLE JERK	120 sec.		60 sec.	L:	R:
	1/2 SNATCH	120 sec.		60 sec.	L:	R:
	HAND 2 HAND SUMO DEADLIFT	30 sec.		60/30/15		
	SIDE BEND (LEFT AND RIGHT)	30 sec.		60/30/15		
	ALTERNATING CLEAN (DIP & SWITCH)	30 sec.		60/30/15		
	FIGURE 8 TO A HOLD	30 sec.		60/30/15		
	CLOSE GRIP PUSH-UP (MILITARY)	30 sec.		60/30/15		

		work time	KB size	rest time	reps	
Round 3	PRESS	120 sec.		60 sec.	L:	R:
	SNATCH	120 sec.		60 sec.	L:	R:
	BEHIND THE NECK SQUAT	30 sec.		60/30/15		
	WINDMILL (LEFT AND RIGHT)	30 sec.		60/30/15		
	DOUBLE KB LONG CYCLE CLEAN	30 sec.		60/30/15		
	STAGGERED PUSH-UP (EXPLOSIVE)	30 sec.		60/30/15		
	HIGH PLANK	30 sec.		60/30/15		

heart rate	comments:
start:	
end:	
5 min. post:	

Im Athletic 6 Month Workout Plan

WARM UP: CHOOSE ONE WARM FROM THE DYNAMIC FLOW DRILL LIST

Round 1

	work time	KB size	rest time	reps	
BOTTOM UP JERK	120 sec.		60 sec.	L:	R:
SNATCH	120 sec.		60 sec.	L:	R:
DOUBLE SQUAT	30 sec.		60/30/15		
BARBELL GET-UP SIT-UP	30 sec.		60/30/15		
DOUBLE KB DEAD CLEAN	30 sec.		60/30/15		
FIGURE 8 TO A HOLD	30 sec.		60/30/15		
PUSH-UP	30 sec.		60/30/15		
PLANK	30 sec.		60/30/15		

Round 2

	work time	KB size	rest time	reps	
LONG CYCLE JERK	120 sec.		60 sec.	L:	R:
1/2 SNATCH	120 sec.		60 sec.	L:	R:
HAND 2 HAND SUMO DEADLIFT	30 sec.		60/30/15		
SIDE BEND (LEFT AND RIGHT)	30 sec.		60/30/15		
ALTERNATING CLEAN (DIP & SWITCH)	30 sec.		60/30/15		
FIGURE 8 TO A HOLD	30 sec.		60/30/15		
CLOSE GRIP PUSH-UP (MILITARY)	30 sec.		60/30/15		

Round 3

	work time	KB size	rest time	reps	
PRESS	120 sec.		60 sec.	L:	R:
SNATCH	120 sec.		60 sec.	L:	R:
BEHIND THE NECK SQUAT	30 sec.		60/30/15		
WINDMILL (LEFT AND RIGHT)	30 sec.		60/30/15		
DOUBLE KB LONG CYCLE CLEAN	30 sec.		60/30/15		
STAGGERED PUSH-UP (EXPLOSIVE)	30 sec.		60/30/15		
HIGH PLANK	30 sec.		60/30/15		

heart rate	comments:
start:	
end:	
5 min. post:	

Im Athletic 6 Month Workout Plan

DATE: _____

WARM UP: CHOOSE ONE WARM FROM THE DYNAMIC FLOW DRILL LIST

Round 1		work time	KB size	rest time	reps	
	BOTTOM UP JERK	120 sec.		60 sec.	L:	R:
	SNATCH	120 sec.		60 sec.	L:	R:
	DOUBLE SQUAT	30 sec.		60/30/15		
	BARBELL GET-UP SIT-UP	30 sec.		60/30/15		
	DOUBLE KB DEAD CLEAN	30 sec.		60/30/15		
	FIGURE 8 TO A HOLD	30 sec.		60/30/15		
	PUSH-UP	30 sec.		60/30/15		
	PLANK	30 sec.		60/30/15		

Round 2		work time	KB size	rest time	reps	
	LONG CYCLE JERK	120 sec.		60 sec.	L:	R:
	1/2 SNATCH	120 sec.		60 sec.	L:	R:
	HAND 2 HAND SUMO DEADLIFT	30 sec.		60/30/15		
	SIDE BEND (LEFT AND RIGHT)	30 sec.		60/30/15		
	ALTERNATING CLEAN (DIP & SWITCH)	30 sec.		60/30/15		
	FIGURE 8 TO A HOLD	30 sec.		60/30/15		
	CLOSE GRIP PUSH-UP (MILITARY)	30 sec.		60/30/15		

Round 3		work time	KB size	rest time	reps	
	PRESS	120 sec.		60 sec.	L:	R:
	SNATCH	120 sec.		60 sec.	L:	R:
	BEHIND THE NECK SQUAT	30 sec.		60/30/15		
	WINDMILL (LEFT AND RIGHT)	30 sec.		60/30/15		
	DOUBLE KB LONG CYCLE CLEAN	30 sec.		60/30/15		
	STAGGERED PUSH-UP (EXPLOSIVE)	30 sec.		60/30/15		
	HIGH PLANK	30 sec.		60/30/15		

heart rate	comments:
start:	
end:	
5 min. post:	

Im Athletic 6 Month Workout Plan

DATE: _____

WARM UP: CHOOSE ONE WARM FROM THE DYNAMIC FLOW DRILL LIST

Round 1		work time	KB size	rest time	reps	
	LONG CYCLE BOTTOM UP PRESS	120 sec.		30 sec.	L:	R:
	SNATCH	120 sec.		30 sec.	L:	R:
	DOUBLE SQUAT	30 sec.		60/30/15		
	BARBELL GET-UP SIT-UP	30 sec.		60/30/15		
	DOUBLE KB DEAD CLEAN	30 sec.		60/30/15		
	FIGURE 8 TO A HOLD	30 sec.		60/30/15		
	PUSH-UP	30 sec.		60/30/15		
	PLANK	30 sec.		60/30/15		

Round 2		work time	KB size	rest time	reps	
	PUSH PRESS	120 sec.		30 sec.	L:	R:
	SNATCH	120 sec.		30 sec.	L:	R:
	HAND 2 HAND SUMO DEADLIFT	30 sec.		60/30/15		
	SIDE BEND (LEFT AND RIGHT)	30 sec.		60/30/15		
	ALTERNATING CLEAN (DIP & SWITCH)	30 sec.		60/30/15		
	FIGURE 8 TO A HOLD	30 sec.		60/30/15		
	CLOSE GRIP PUSH-UP (MILITARY)	30 sec.		60/30/15		

Round 3		work time	KB size	rest time	reps	
	LONG CYCLE JERK	120 sec.		30 sec.	L:	R:
	SNATCH	120 sec.		30 sec.	L:	R:
	BEHIND THE NECK SQUAT	30 sec.		60/30/15		
	WINDMILL (LEFT AND RIGHT)	30 sec.		60/30/15		
	DOUBLE KB LONG CYCLE CLEAN	30 sec.		60/30/15		
	STAGGERED PUSH-UP (EXPLOSIVE)	30 sec.		60/30/15		
	HIGH PLANK	30 sec.		60/30/15		

heart rate	comments:
start:	
end:	
5 min. post:	

Im Athletic 6 Month Workout Plan

DATE: _____

WARM UP: CHOOSE ONE WARM FROM THE DYNAMIC FLOW DRILL LIST

		work time	KB size	rest time	reps	
Round 1	LONG CYCLE BOTTOM UP PRESS	120 sec.		30 sec.	L:	R:
	SNATCH	120 sec.		30 sec.	L:	R:
	DOUBLE SQUAT	30 sec.		60/30/15		
	BARBELL GET-UP SIT-UP	30 sec.		60/30/15		
	DOUBLE KB DEAD CLEAN	30 sec.		60/30/15		
	FIGURE 8 TO A HOLD	30 sec.		60/30/15		
	PUSH-UP	30 sec.		60/30/15		
	PLANK	30 sec.		60/30/15		

		work time	KB size	rest time	reps	
Round 2	PUSH PRESS	120 sec.		30 sec.	L:	R:
	SNATCH	120 sec.		30 sec.	L:	R:
	HAND 2 HAND SUMO DEADLIFT	30 sec.		60/30/15		
	SIDE BEND (LEFT AND RIGHT)	30 sec.		60/30/15		
	ALTERNATING CLEAN (DIP & SWITCH)	30 sec.		60/30/15		
	FIGURE 8 TO A HOLD	30 sec.		60/30/15		
	CLOSE GRIP PUSH-UP (MILITARY)	30 sec.		60/30/15		

		work time	KB size	rest time	reps	
Round 3	LONG CYCLE JERK	120 sec.		30 sec.	L:	R:
	SNATCH	120 sec.		30 sec.	L:	R:
	BEHIND THE NECK SQUAT	30 sec.		60/30/15		
	WINDMILL (LEFT AND RIGHT)	30 sec.		60/30/15		
	DOUBLE KB LONG CYCLE CLEAN	30 sec.		60/30/15		
	STAGGERED PUSH-UP (EXPLOSIVE)	30 sec.		60/30/15		
	HIGH PLANK	30 sec.		60/30/15		

heart rate	comments:
start:	
end:	
5 min. post:	

Im Athletic 6 Month Workout Plan

DATE: _____

WARM UP: CHOOSE ONE WARM FROM THE DYNAMIC FLOW DRILL LIST

Round 1		work time	KB size	rest time	reps	
	LONG CYCLE BOTTOM UP PRESS	120 sec.		30 sec.	L:	R:
	SNATCH	120 sec.		30 sec.	L:	R:
	DOUBLE SQUAT	30 sec.		60/30/15		
	BARBELL GET-UP SIT-UP	30 sec.		60/30/15		
	DOUBLE KB DEAD CLEAN	30 sec.		60/30/15		
	FIGURE 8 TO A HOLD	30 sec.		60/30/15		
	PUSH-UP	30 sec.		60/30/15		
	PLANK	30 sec.		60/30/15		

Round 2		work time	KB size	rest time	reps	
	PUSH PRESS	120 sec.		30 sec.	L:	R:
	SNATCH	120 sec.		30 sec.	L:	R:
	HAND 2 HAND SUMO DEADLIFT	30 sec.		60/30/15		
	SIDE BEND (LEFT AND RIGHT)	30 sec.		60/30/15		
	ALTERNATING CLEAN (DIP & SWITCH)	30 sec.		60/30/15		
	FIGURE 8 TO A HOLD	30 sec.		60/30/15		
	CLOSE GRIP PUSH-UP (MILITARY)	30 sec.		60/30/15		

Round 3		work time	KB size	rest time	reps	
	LONG CYCLE JERK	120 sec.		30 sec.	L:	R:
	SNATCH	120 sec.		30 sec.	L:	R:
	BEHIND THE NECK SQUAT	30 sec.		60/30/15		
	WINDMILL (LEFT AND RIGHT)	30 sec.		60/30/15		
	DOUBLE KB LONG CYCLE CLEAN	30 sec.		60/30/15		
	STAGGERED PUSH-UP (EXPLOSIVE)	30 sec.		60/30/15		
	HIGH PLANK	30 sec.		60/30/15		

heart rate	comments:
start:	
end:	
5 min. post:	

Im Athletic 6 Month Workout Plan

DATE: _____

WARM UP: CHOOSE ONE WARM FROM THE DYNAMIC FLOW DRILL LIST

Round 1		work time	KB size	rest time	reps	
	LONG CYCLE BOTTOM UP PRESS	120 sec.		30 sec.	L:	R:
	SNATCH	120 sec.		30 sec.	L:	R:
	DOUBLE SQUAT	30 sec.		60/30/15		
	BARBELL GET-UP SIT-UP	30 sec.		60/30/15		
	DOUBLE KB DEAD CLEAN	30 sec.		60/30/15		
	FIGURE 8 TO A HOLD	30 sec.		60/30/15		
	PUSH-UP	30 sec.		60/30/15		
	PLANK	30 sec.		60/30/15		

Round 2		work time	KB size	rest time	reps	
	PUSH PRESS	120 sec.		30 sec.	L:	R:
	SNATCH	120 sec.		30 sec.	L:	R:
	HAND 2 HAND SUMO DEADLIFT	30 sec.		60/30/15		
	SIDE BEND (LEFT AND RIGHT)	30 sec.		60/30/15		
	ALTERNATING CLEAN (DIP & SWITCH)	30 sec.		60/30/15		
	FIGURE 8 TO A HOLD	30 sec.		60/30/15		
	CLOSE GRIP PUSH-UP (MILITARY)	30 sec.		60/30/15		

Round 3		work time	KB size	rest time	reps	
	LONG CYCLE JERK	120 sec.		30 sec.	L:	R:
	SNATCH	120 sec.		30 sec.	L:	R:
	BEHIND THE NECK SQUAT	30 sec.		60/30/15		
	WINDMILL (LEFT AND RIGHT)	30 sec.		60/30/15		
	DOUBLE KB LONG CYCLE CLEAN	30 sec.		60/30/15		
	STAGGERED PUSH-UP (EXPLOSIVE)	30 sec.		60/30/15		
	HIGH PLANK	30 sec.		60/30/15		

heart rate	comments:
start:	
end:	
5 min. post:	

You've finished month 5!

"I've got a theory that if you give 100 percent all of the time, somehow things will work out in the end." – Larry Bird

Im Athletic 6 Month Workout Plan

DATE: _____

WARM UP: CHOOSE ONE WARM FROM THE DYNAMIC FLOW DRILL LIST

		work time	KB size	rest time	reps	
Round 1	JERK	180 sec.		120 sec.	L:	R:
	SNATCH	180 sec.		120 sec.	L:	R:
	DOUBLE SQUAT	30 sec.		60/30/15		
	BARBELL GET-UP SIT-UP	30 sec.		60/30/15		
	DOUBLE KB DEAD CLEAN	30 sec.		60/30/15		
	FIGURE 8 TO A HOLD	30 sec.		60/30/15		
	PUSH-UP	30 sec.		60/30/15		
	PLANK	30 sec.		60/30/15		

		work time	KB size	rest time	reps	
Round 2	LONG CYCLE JERK	180 sec.		120 sec.	L:	R:
	1/2 SNATCH	180 sec.		120 sec.	L:	R:
	HAND 2 HAND SUMO DEADLIFT	30 sec.		60/30/15		
	SIDE BEND (LEFT AND RIGHT)	30 sec.		60/30/15		
	ALTERNATING CLEAN (DIP & SWITCH)	30 sec.		60/30/15		
	FIGURE 8 TO A HOLD	30 sec.		60/30/15		
	CLOSE GRIP PUSH-UP (MILITARY)	30 sec.		60/30/15		

		work time	KB size	rest time	reps	
Round 3	PRESS	180 sec.		120 sec.	L:	R:
	SNATCH	180 sec.		120 sec.	L:	R:
	BEHIND THE NECK SQUAT	30 sec.		60/30/15		
	WINDMILL (LEFT AND RIGHT)	30 sec.		60/30/15		
	DOUBLE KB LONG CYCLE CLEAN	30 sec.		60/30/15		
	STAGGERED PUSH-UP (EXPLOSIVE)	30 sec.		60/30/15		
	HIGH PLANK	30 sec.		60/30/15		

heart rate	comments:
start:	
end:	
5 min. post:	

Im Athletic 6 Month Workout Plan

DATE: _____

WARM UP: CHOOSE ONE WARM FROM THE DYNAMIC FLOW DRILL LIST

Round 1

	work time	KB size	rest time	reps	
JERK	180 sec.		120 sec.	L:	R:
SNATCH	180 sec.		120 sec.	L:	R:
DOUBLE SQUAT	30 sec.		60/30/15		
BARBELL GET-UP SIT-UP	30 sec.		60/30/15		
DOUBLE KB DEAD CLEAN	30 sec.		60/30/15		
FIGURE 8 TO A HOLD	30 sec.		60/30/15		
PUSH-UP	30 sec.		60/30/15		
PLANK	30 sec.		60/30/15		

Round 2

	work time	KB size	rest time	reps	
LONG CYCLE JERK	180 sec.		120 sec.	L:	R:
1/2 SNATCH	180 sec.		120 sec.	L:	R:
HAND 2 HAND SUMO DEADLIFT	30 sec.		60/30/15		
SIDE BEND (LEFT AND RIGHT)	30 sec.		60/30/15		
ALTERNATING CLEAN (DIP & SWITCH)	30 sec.		60/30/15		
FIGURE 8 TO A HOLD	30 sec.		60/30/15		
CLOSE GRIP PUSH-UP (MILITARY)	30 sec.		60/30/15		

Round 3

	work time	KB size	rest time	reps	
PRESS	180 sec.		120 sec.	L:	R:
SNATCH	180 sec.		120 sec.	L:	R:
BEHIND THE NECK SQUAT	30 sec.		60/30/15		
WINDMILL (LEFT AND RIGHT)	30 sec.		60/30/15		
DOUBLE KB LONG CYCLE CLEAN	30 sec.		60/30/15		
STAGGERED PUSH-UP (EXPLOSIVE)	30 sec.		60/30/15		
HIGH PLANK	30 sec.		60/30/15		

heart rate	comments:
start:	
end:	
5 min. post:	

Im Athletic 6 Month Workout Plan

DATE: _____

WARM UP: CHOOSE ONE WARM FROM THE DYNAMIC FLOW DRILL LIST

		work time	KB size	rest time	reps	
Round 1	JERK	180 sec.		120 sec.	L:	R:
	SNATCH	180 sec.		120 sec.	L:	R:
	DOUBLE SQUAT	30 sec.		60/30/15		
	BARBELL GET-UP SIT-UP	30 sec.		60/30/15		
	DOUBLE KB DEAD CLEAN	30 sec.		60/30/15		
	FIGURE 8 TO A HOLD	30 sec.		60/30/15		
	PUSH-UP	30 sec.		60/30/15		
	PLANK	30 sec.		60/30/15		

		work time	KB size	rest time	reps	
Round 2	LONG CYCLE JERK	180 sec.		120 sec.	L:	R:
	1/2 SNATCH	180 sec.		120 sec.	L:	R:
	HAND 2 HAND SUMO DEADLIFT	30 sec.		60/30/15		
	SIDE BEND (LEFT AND RIGHT)	30 sec.		60/30/15		
	ALTERNATING CLEAN (DIP & SWITCH)	30 sec.		60/30/15		
	FIGURE 8 TO A HOLD	30 sec.		60/30/15		
	CLOSE GRIP PUSH-UP (MILITARY)	30 sec.		60/30/15		

		work time	KB size	rest time	reps	
Round 3	PRESS	180 sec.		120 sec.	L:	R:
	SNATCH	180 sec.		120 sec.	L:	R:
	BEHIND THE NECK SQUAT	30 sec.		60/30/15		
	WINDMILL (LEFT AND RIGHT)	30 sec.		60/30/15		
	DOUBLE KB LONG CYCLE CLEAN	30 sec.		60/30/15		
	STAGGERED PUSH-UP (EXPLOSIVE)	30 sec.		60/30/15		
	HIGH PLANK	30 sec.		60/30/15		

heart rate	comments:
start:	
end:	
5 min. post:	

Im Athletic 6 Month Workout Plan

DATE: _____

WARM UP: CHOOSE ONE WARM FROM THE DYNAMIC FLOW DRILL LIST

		work time	KB size	rest time	reps	
Round 1	JERK	180 sec.		120 sec.	L:	R:
	SNATCH	180 sec.		120 sec.	L:	R:
	DOUBLE SQUAT	30 sec.		60/30/15		
	BARBELL GET-UP SIT-UP	30 sec.		60/30/15		
	DOUBLE KB DEAD CLEAN	30 sec.		60/30/15		
	FIGURE 8 TO A HOLD	30 sec.		60/30/15		
	PUSH-UP	30 sec.		60/30/15		
	PLANK	30 sec.		60/30/15		

		work time	KB size	rest time	reps	
Round 2	LONG CYCLE JERK	180 sec.		120 sec.	L:	R:
	1/2 SNATCH	180 sec.		120 sec.	L:	R:
	HAND 2 HAND SUMO DEADLIFT	30 sec.		60/30/15		
	SIDE BEND (LEFT AND RIGHT)	30 sec.		60/30/15		
	ALTERNATING CLEAN (DIP & SWITCH)	30 sec.		60/30/15		
	FIGURE 8 TO A HOLD	30 sec.		60/30/15		
	CLOSE GRIP PUSH-UP (MILITARY)	30 sec.		60/30/15		

		work time	KB size	rest time	reps	
Round 3	PRESS	180 sec.		120 sec.	L:	R:
	SNATCH	180 sec.		120 sec.	L:	R:
	BEHIND THE NECK SQUAT	30 sec.		60/30/15		
	WINDMILL (LEFT AND RIGHT)	30 sec.		60/30/15		
	DOUBLE KB LONG CYCLE CLEAN	30 sec.		60/30/15		
	STAGGERED PUSH-UP (EXPLOSIVE)	30 sec.		60/30/15		
	HIGH PLANK	30 sec.		60/30/15		

heart rate	comments:
start:	
end:	
5 min. post:	

Im Athletic 6 Month Workout Plan

DATE: _____

WARM UP: CHOOSE ONE WARM FROM THE DYNAMIC FLOW DRILL LIST

		work time	KB size	rest time	reps	
Round 1	LONG CYCLE BOTTOM UP PRESS	180 sec.		90 sec.	L:	R:
	1/2 SNATCH	180 sec.		90 sec.	L:	R:
	DOUBLE SQUAT	30 sec.		60/30/15		
	BARBELL GET-UP SIT-UP	30 sec.		60/30/15		
	DOUBLE KB DEAD CLEAN	30 sec.		60/30/15		
	FIGURE 8 TO A HOLD	30 sec.		60/30/15		
	PUSH-UP	30 sec.		60/30/15		
	PLANK	30 sec.		60/30/15		

		work time	KB size	rest time	reps	
Round 2	JERK	180 sec.		90 sec.	L:	R:
	SNATCH	180 sec.		90 sec.	L:	R:
	HAND 2 HAND SUMO DEADLIFT	30 sec.		60/30/15		
	SIDE BEND (LEFT AND RIGHT)	30 sec.		60/30/15		
	ALTERNATING CLEAN (DIP & SWITCH)	30 sec.		60/30/15		
	FIGURE 8 TO A HOLD	30 sec.		60/30/15		
	CLOSE GRIP PUSH-UP (MILITARY)	30 sec.		60/30/15		

		work time	KB size	rest time	reps	
Round 3	PRESS	180 sec.		90 sec.	L:	R:
	SNATCH	180 sec.		90 sec.	L:	R:
	BEHIND THE NECK SQUAT	30 sec.		60/30/15		
	WINDMILL (LEFT AND RIGHT)	30 sec.		60/30/15		
	DOUBLE KB LONG CYCLE CLEAN	30 sec.		60/30/15		
	STAGGERED PUSH-UP (EXPLOSIVE)	30 sec.		60/30/15		
	HIGH PLANK	30 sec.		60/30/15		

heart rate	comments:
start:	
end:	
5 min. post:	

Im Athletic 6 Month Workout Plan

DATE: _____

WARM UP: CHOOSE ONE WARM FROM THE DYNAMIC FLOW DRILL LIST

		work time	KB size	rest time	reps	
Round 1	LONG CYCLE BOTTOM UP PRESS	180 sec.		90 sec.	L:	R:
	1/2 SNATCH	180 sec.		90 sec.	L:	R:
	DOUBLE SQUAT	30 sec.		60/30/15		
	BARBELL GET-UP SIT-UP	30 sec.		60/30/15		
	DOUBLE KB DEAD CLEAN	30 sec.		60/30/15		
	FIGURE 8 TO A HOLD	30 sec.		60/30/15		
	PUSH-UP	30 sec.		60/30/15		
	PLANK	30 sec.		60/30/15		

		work time	KB size	rest time	reps	
Round 2	JERK	180 sec.		90 sec.	L:	R:
	SNATCH	180 sec.		90 sec.	L:	R:
	HAND 2 HAND SUMO DEADLIFT	30 sec.		60/30/15		
	SIDE BEND (LEFT AND RIGHT)	30 sec.		60/30/15		
	ALTERNATING CLEAN (DIP & SWITCH)	30 sec.		60/30/15		
	FIGURE 8 TO A HOLD	30 sec.		60/30/15		
	CLOSE GRIP PUSH-UP (MILITARY)	30 sec.		60/30/15		

		work time	KB size	rest time	reps	
Round 3	PRESS	180 sec.		90 sec.	L:	R:
	SNATCH	180 sec.		90 sec.	L:	R:
	BEHIND THE NECK SQUAT	30 sec.		60/30/15		
	WINDMILL (LEFT AND RIGHT)	30 sec.		60/30/15		
	DOUBLE KB LONG CYCLE CLEAN	30 sec.		60/30/15		
	STAGGERED PUSH-UP (EXPLOSIVE)	30 sec.		60/30/15		
	HIGH PLANK	30 sec.		60/30/15		

heart rate	comments:
start:	
end:	
5 min. post:	

Im Athletic 6 Month Workout Plan

DATE: _____

WARM UP: CHOOSE ONE WARM FROM THE DYNAMIC FLOW DRILL LIST

Round 1		work time	KB size	rest time	reps	
	LONG CYCLE BOTTOM UP PRESS	180 sec.		90 sec.	L:	R:
	1/2 SNATCH	180 sec.		90 sec.	L:	R:
	DOUBLE SQUAT	30 sec.		60/30/15		
	BARBELL GET-UP SIT-UP	30 sec.		60/30/15		
	DOUBLE KB DEAD CLEAN	30 sec.		60/30/15		
	FIGURE 8 TO A HOLD	30 sec.		60/30/15		
	PUSH-UP	30 sec.		60/30/15		
	PLANK	30 sec.		60/30/15		

Round 2		work time	KB size	rest time	reps	
	JERK	180 sec.		90 sec.	L:	R:
	SNATCH	180 sec.		90 sec.	L:	R:
	HAND 2 HAND SUMO DEADLIFT	30 sec.		60/30/15		
	SIDE BEND (LEFT AND RIGHT)	30 sec.		60/30/15		
	ALTERNATING CLEAN (DIP & SWITCH)	30 sec.		60/30/15		
	FIGURE 8 TO A HOLD	30 sec.		60/30/15		
	CLOSE GRIP PUSH-UP (MILITARY)	30 sec.		60/30/15		

Round 3		work time	KB size	rest time	reps	
	PRESS	180 sec.		90 sec.	L:	R:
	SNATCH	180 sec.		90 sec.	L:	R:
	BEHIND THE NECK SQUAT	30 sec.		60/30/15		
	WINDMILL (LEFT AND RIGHT)	30 sec.		60/30/15		
	DOUBLE KB LONG CYCLE CLEAN	30 sec.		60/30/15		
	STAGGERED PUSH-UP (EXPLOSIVE)	30 sec.		60/30/15		
	HIGH PLANK	30 sec.		60/30/15		

heart rate	comments:
start:	
end:	
5 min. post:	

Im Athletic 6 Month Workout Plan

DATE: _____

WARM UP: CHOOSE ONE WARM FROM THE DYNAMIC FLOW DRILL LIST

Round	Exercise	work time	KB size	rest time	reps	
Round 1	LONG CYCLE BOTTOM UP PRESS	180 sec.		90 sec.	L:	R:
	1/2 SNATCH	180 sec.		90 sec.	L:	R:
	DOUBLE SQUAT	30 sec.		60/30/15		
	BARBELL GET-UP SIT-UP	30 sec.		60/30/15		
	DOUBLE KB DEAD CLEAN	30 sec.		60/30/15		
	FIGURE 8 TO A HOLD	30 sec.		60/30/15		
	PUSH-UP	30 sec.		60/30/15		
	PLANK	30 sec.		60/30/15		

Round	Exercise	work time	KB size	rest time	reps	
Round 2	JERK	180 sec.		90 sec.	L:	R:
	SNATCH	180 sec.		90 sec.	L:	R:
	HAND 2 HAND SUMO DEADLIFT	30 sec.		60/30/15		
	SIDE BEND (LEFT AND RIGHT)	30 sec.		60/30/15		
	ALTERNATING CLEAN (DIP & SWITCH)	30 sec.		60/30/15		
	FIGURE 8 TO A HOLD	30 sec.		60/30/15		
	CLOSE GRIP PUSH-UP (MILITARY)	30 sec.		60/30/15		

Round	Exercise	work time	KB size	rest time	reps	
Round 3	PRESS	180 sec.		90 sec.	L:	R:
	SNATCH	180 sec.		90 sec.	L:	R:
	BEHIND THE NECK SQUAT	30 sec.		60/30/15		
	WINDMILL (LEFT AND RIGHT)	30 sec.		60/30/15		
	DOUBLE KB LONG CYCLE CLEAN	30 sec.		60/30/15		
	STAGGERED PUSH-UP (EXPLOSIVE)	30 sec.		60/30/15		
	HIGH PLANK	30 sec.		60/30/15		

heart rate	comments:
start:	
end:	
5 min. post:	

Im Athletic 6 Month Workout Plan

WARM UP: CHOOSE ONE WARM FROM THE DYNAMIC FLOW DRILL LIST

		work time	KB size	rest time	reps	
Round 1	LONG CYCLE JERK	180 sec.		60 sec.	L:	R:
	1/2 SNATCH	180 sec.		60 sec.	L:	R:
	DOUBLE SQUAT	30 sec.		60/30/15		
	BARBELL GET-UP SIT-UP	30 sec.		60/30/15		
	DOUBLE KB DEAD CLEAN	30 sec.		60/30/15		
	FIGURE 8 TO A HOLD	30 sec.		60/30/15		
	PUSH-UP	30 sec.		60/30/15		
	PLANK	30 sec.		60/30/15		

		work time	KB size	rest time	reps	
Round 2	JERK	180 sec.		60 sec.	L:	R:
	SNATCH	180 sec.		60 sec.	L:	R:
	HAND 2 HAND SUMO DEADLIFT	30 sec.		60/30/15		
	SIDE BEND (LEFT AND RIGHT)	30 sec.		60/30/15		
	ALTERNATING CLEAN (DIP & SWITCH)	30 sec.		60/30/15		
	FIGURE 8 TO A HOLD	30 sec.		60/30/15		
	CLOSE GRIP PUSH-UP (MILITARY)	30 sec.		60/30/15		

		work time	KB size	rest time	reps	
Round 3	LONG CYCLE JERK	180 sec.		60 sec.	L:	R:
	1/2 SNATCH	180 sec.		60 sec.	L:	R:
	BEHIND THE NECK SQUAT	30 sec.		60/30/15		
	WINDMILL (LEFT AND RIGHT)	30 sec.		60/30/15		
	DOUBLE KB LONG CYCLE CLEAN	30 sec.		60/30/15		
	STAGGERED PUSH-UP (EXPLOSIVE)	30 sec.		60/30/15		
	HIGH PLANK	30 sec.		60/30/15		

heart rate	comments:
start:	
end:	
5 min. post:	

Im Athletic 6 Month Workout Plan

WARM UP: CHOOSE ONE WARM FROM THE DYNAMIC FLOW DRILL LIST

Round 1

	work time	KB size	rest time	reps	
LONG CYCLE JERK	180 sec.		60 sec.	L:	R:
1/2 SNATCH	180 sec.		60 sec.	L:	R:
DOUBLE SQUAT	30 sec.		60/30/15		
BARBELL GET-UP SIT-UP	30 sec.		60/30/15		
DOUBLE KB DEAD CLEAN	30 sec.		60/30/15		
FIGURE 8 TO A HOLD	30 sec.		60/30/15		
PUSH-UP	30 sec.		60/30/15		
PLANK	30 sec.		60/30/15		

Round 2

	work time	KB size	rest time	reps	
JERK	180 sec.		60 sec.	L:	R:
SNATCH	180 sec.		60 sec.	L:	R:
HAND 2 HAND SUMO DEADLIFT	30 sec.		60/30/15		
SIDE BEND (LEFT AND RIGHT)	30 sec.		60/30/15		
ALTERNATING CLEAN (DIP & SWITCH)	30 sec.		60/30/15		
FIGURE 8 TO A HOLD	30 sec.		60/30/15		
CLOSE GRIP PUSH-UP (MILITARY)	30 sec.		60/30/15		

Round 3

	work time	KB size	rest time	reps	
LONG CYCLE JERK	180 sec.		60 sec.	L:	R:
1/2 SNATCH	180 sec.		60 sec.	L:	R:
BEHIND THE NECK SQUAT	30 sec.		60/30/15		
WINDMILL (LEFT AND RIGHT)	30 sec.		60/30/15		
DOUBLE KB LONG CYCLE CLEAN	30 sec.		60/30/15		
STAGGERED PUSH-UP (EXPLOSIVE)	30 sec.		60/30/15		
HIGH PLANK	30 sec.		60/30/15		

heart rate	comments:
start:	
end:	
5 min. post:	

Im Athletic 6 Month Workout Plan

DATE: _____

MONTH: 6
WEEK: 3
DAY: 3

WARM UP: CHOOSE ONE WARM FROM THE DYNAMIC FLOW DRILL LIST

		work time	KB size	rest time	reps	
Round 1	LONG CYCLE JERK	180 sec.		60 sec.	L:	R:
	1/2 SNATCH	180 sec.		60 sec.	L:	R:
	DOUBLE SQUAT	30 sec.		60/30/15		
	BARBELL GET-UP SIT-UP	30 sec.		60/30/15		
	DOUBLE KB DEAD CLEAN	30 sec.		60/30/15		
	FIGURE 8 TO A HOLD	30 sec.		60/30/15		
	PUSH-UP	30 sec.		60/30/15		
	PLANK	30 sec.		60/30/15		

		work time	KB size	rest time	reps	
Round 2	JERK	180 sec.		60 sec.	L:	R:
	SNATCH	180 sec.		60 sec.	L:	R:
	HAND 2 HAND SUMO DEADLIFT	30 sec.		60/30/15		
	SIDE BEND (LEFT AND RIGHT)	30 sec.		60/30/15		
	ALTERNATING CLEAN (DIP & SWITCH)	30 sec.		60/30/15		
	FIGURE 8 TO A HOLD	30 sec.		60/30/15		
	CLOSE GRIP PUSH-UP (MILITARY)	30 sec.		60/30/15		

		work time	KB size	rest time	reps	
Round 3	LONG CYCLE JERK	180 sec.		60 sec.	L:	R:
	1/2 SNATCH	180 sec.		60 sec.	L:	R:
	BEHIND THE NECK SQUAT	30 sec.		60/30/15		
	WINDMILL (LEFT AND RIGHT)	30 sec.		60/30/15		
	DOUBLE KB LONG CYCLE CLEAN	30 sec.		60/30/15		
	STAGGERED PUSH-UP (EXPLOSIVE)	30 sec.		60/30/15		
	HIGH PLANK	30 sec.		60/30/15		

heart rate	comments:
start:	
end:	
5 min. post:	

Im Athletic 6 Month Workout Plan

DATE: _____

WARM UP: CHOOSE ONE WARM FROM THE DYNAMIC FLOW DRILL LIST

Round 1		work time	KB size	rest time	reps	
	LONG CYCLE JERK	180 sec.		60 sec.	L:	R:
	1/2 SNATCH	180 sec.		60 sec.	L:	R:
	DOUBLE SQUAT	30 sec.		60/30/15		
	BARBELL GET-UP SIT-UP	30 sec.		60/30/15		
	DOUBLE KB DEAD CLEAN	30 sec.		60/30/15		
	FIGURE 8 TO A HOLD	30 sec.		60/30/15		
	PUSH-UP	30 sec.		60/30/15		
	PLANK	30 sec.		60/30/15		

Round 2		work time	KB size	rest time	reps	
	JERK	180 sec.		60 sec.	L:	R:
	SNATCH	180 sec.		60 sec.	L:	R:
	HAND 2 HAND SUMO DEADLIFT	30 sec.		60/30/15		
	SIDE BEND (LEFT AND RIGHT)	30 sec.		60/30/15		
	ALTERNATING CLEAN (DIP & SWITCH)	30 sec.		60/30/15		
	FIGURE 8 TO A HOLD	30 sec.		60/30/15		
	CLOSE GRIP PUSH-UP (MILITARY)	30 sec.		60/30/15		

Round 3		work time	KB size	rest time	reps	
	LONG CYCLE JERK	180 sec.		60 sec.	L:	R:
	1/2 SNATCH	180 sec.		60 sec.	L:	R:
	BEHIND THE NECK SQUAT	30 sec.		60/30/15		
	WINDMILL (LEFT AND RIGHT)	30 sec.		60/30/15		
	DOUBLE KB LONG CYCLE CLEAN	30 sec.		60/30/15		
	STAGGERED PUSH-UP (EXPLOSIVE)	30 sec.		60/30/15		
	HIGH PLANK	30 sec.		60/30/15		

heart rate	comments:
start:	
end:	
5 min. post:	

Im Athletic 6 Month Workout Plan

DATE: _____

MONTH: 6
WEEK: 4
DAY: 1

WARM UP: CHOOSE ONE WARM FROM THE DYNAMIC FLOW DRILL LIST

		work time	KB size	rest time	reps	
Round 1	PRESS	180 sec.		30 sec.	L:	R:
	SNATCH	180 sec.		30 sec.	L:	R:
	DOUBLE SQUAT	30 sec.		60/30/15		
	BARBELL GET-UP SIT-UP	30 sec.		60/30/15		
	DOUBLE KB DEAD CLEAN	30 sec.		60/30/15		
	FIGURE 8 TO A HOLD	30 sec.		60/30/15		
	PUSH-UP	30 sec.		60/30/15		
	PLANK	30 sec.		60/30/15		

		work time	KB size	rest time	reps	
Round 2	JERK	180 sec.		30 sec.	L:	R:
	SNATCH	180 sec.		30 sec.	L:	R:
	HAND 2 HAND SUMO DEADLIFT	30 sec.		60/30/15		
	SIDE BEND (LEFT AND RIGHT)	30 sec.		60/30/15		
	ALTERNATING CLEAN (DIP & SWITCH)	30 sec.		60/30/15		
	FIGURE 8 TO A HOLD	30 sec.		60/30/15		
	CLOSE GRIP PUSH-UP (MILITARY)	30 sec.		60/30/15		

		work time	KB size	rest time	reps	
Round 3	LONG CYCLE JERK	180 sec.		30 sec.	L:	R:
	SNATCH	180 sec.		30 sec.	L:	R:
	BEHIND THE NECK SQUAT	30 sec.		60/30/15		
	WINDMILL (LEFT AND RIGHT)	30 sec.		60/30/15		
	DOUBLE KB LONG CYCLE CLEAN	30 sec.		60/30/15		
	STAGGERED PUSH-UP (EXPLOSIVE)	30 sec.		60/30/15		
	HIGH PLANK	30 sec.		60/30/15		

heart rate	comments:
start:	
end:	
5 min. post:	

Im Athletic 6 Month Workout Plan

WARM UP: CHOOSE ONE WARM FROM THE DYNAMIC FLOW DRILL LIST

		work time	KB size	rest time	reps	
Round 1	PRESS	180 sec.		30 sec.	L:	R:
	SNATCH	180 sec.		30 sec.	L:	R:
	DOUBLE SQUAT	30 sec.		60/30/15		
	BARBELL GET-UP SIT-UP	30 sec.		60/30/15		
	DOUBLE KB DEAD CLEAN	30 sec.		60/30/15		
	FIGURE 8 TO A HOLD	30 sec.		60/30/15		
	PUSH-UP	30 sec.		60/30/15		
	PLANK	30 sec.		60/30/15		

		work time	KB size	rest time	reps	
Round 2	JERK	180 sec.		30 sec.	L:	R:
	SNATCH	180 sec.		30 sec.	L:	R:
	HAND 2 HAND SUMO DEADLIFT	30 sec.		60/30/15		
	SIDE BEND (LEFT AND RIGHT)	30 sec.		60/30/15		
	ALTERNATING CLEAN (DIP & SWITCH)	30 sec.		60/30/15		
	FIGURE 8 TO A HOLD	30 sec.		60/30/15		
	CLOSE GRIP PUSH-UP (MILITARY)	30 sec.		60/30/15		

		work time	KB size	rest time	reps	
Round 3	LONG CYCLE JERK	180 sec.		30 sec.	L:	R:
	SNATCH	180 sec.		30 sec.	L:	R:
	BEHIND THE NECK SQUAT	30 sec.		60/30/15		
	WINDMILL (LEFT AND RIGHT)	30 sec.		60/30/15		
	DOUBLE KB LONG CYCLE CLEAN	30 sec.		60/30/15		
	STAGGERED PUSH-UP (EXPLOSIVE)	30 sec.		60/30/15		
	HIGH PLANK	30 sec.		60/30/15		

heart rate	comments:
start:	
end:	
5 min. post:	

Im Athletic 6 Month Workout Plan

DATE: _____

WARM UP: CHOOSE ONE WARM FROM THE DYNAMIC FLOW DRILL LIST

		work time	KB size	rest time	reps	
Round 1	PRESS	180 sec.		30 sec.	L:	R:
	SNATCH	180 sec.		30 sec.	L:	R:
	DOUBLE SQUAT	30 sec.		60/30/15		
	BARBELL GET-UP SIT-UP	30 sec.		60/30/15		
	DOUBLE KB DEAD CLEAN	30 sec.		60/30/15		
	FIGURE 8 TO A HOLD	30 sec.		60/30/15		
	PUSH-UP	30 sec.		60/30/15		
	PLANK	30 sec.		60/30/15		

		work time	KB size	rest time	reps	
Round 2	JERK	180 sec.		30 sec.	L:	R:
	SNATCH	180 sec.		30 sec.	L:	R:
	HAND 2 HAND SUMO DEADLIFT	30 sec.		60/30/15		
	SIDE BEND (LEFT AND RIGHT)	30 sec.		60/30/15		
	ALTERNATING CLEAN (DIP & SWITCH)	30 sec.		60/30/15		
	FIGURE 8 TO A HOLD	30 sec.		60/30/15		
	CLOSE GRIP PUSH-UP (MILITARY)	30 sec.		60/30/15		

		work time	KB size	rest time	reps	
Round 3	LONG CYCLE JERK	180 sec.		30 sec.	L:	R:
	SNATCH	180 sec.		30 sec.	L:	R:
	BEHIND THE NECK SQUAT	30 sec.		60/30/15		
	WINDMILL (LEFT AND RIGHT)	30 sec.		60/30/15		
	DOUBLE KB LONG CYCLE CLEAN	30 sec.		60/30/15		
	STAGGERED PUSH-UP (EXPLOSIVE)	30 sec.		60/30/15		
	HIGH PLANK	30 sec.		60/30/15		

heart rate	comments:
start:	
end:	
5 min. post:	

Im Athletic 6 Month Workout Plan

DATE: _____

WARM UP: CHOOSE ONE WARM FROM THE DYNAMIC FLOW DRILL LIST

		work time	KB size	rest time	reps	
Round 1	PRESS	180 sec.		30 sec.	L:	R:
	SNATCH	180 sec.		30 sec.	L:	R:
	DOUBLE SQUAT	30 sec.		60/30/15		
	BARBELL GET-UP SIT-UP	30 sec.		60/30/15		
	DOUBLE KB DEAD CLEAN	30 sec.		60/30/15		
	FIGURE 8 TO A HOLD	30 sec.		60/30/15		
	PUSH-UP	30 sec.		60/30/15		
	PLANK	30 sec.		60/30/15		

		work time	KB size	rest time	reps	
Round 2	JERK	180 sec.		30 sec.	L:	R:
	SNATCH	180 sec.		30 sec.	L:	R:
	HAND 2 HAND SUMO DEADLIFT	30 sec.		60/30/15		
	SIDE BEND (LEFT AND RIGHT)	30 sec.		60/30/15		
	ALTERNATING CLEAN (DIP & SWITCH)	30 sec.		60/30/15		
	FIGURE 8 TO A HOLD	30 sec.		60/30/15		
	CLOSE GRIP PUSH-UP (MILITARY)	30 sec.		60/30/15		

		work time	KB size	rest time	reps	
Round 3	LONG CYCLE JERK	180 sec.		30 sec.	L:	R:
	SNATCH	180 sec.		30 sec.	L:	R:
	BEHIND THE NECK SQUAT	30 sec.		60/30/15		
	WINDMILL (LEFT AND RIGHT)	30 sec.		60/30/15		
	DOUBLE KB LONG CYCLE CLEAN	30 sec.		60/30/15		
	STAGGERED PUSH-UP (EXPLOSIVE)	30 sec.		60/30/15		
	HIGH PLANK	30 sec.		60/30/15		

heart rate	comments:
start:	
end:	
5 min. post:	

Benefit No. 3 to Kettlebell training:

Acceleration and Deceleration training: Kettlebell drills provide intense acceleration to many of the core muscle groups such as the hips and glutes. This acceleration transfers to many athletic skills such as jumping running, and throwing. Inversely, deceleration occurs at the end of the kettlebell movement transferring that strength into your core.

Congratulations. You've come to the end of the 6 month program. By now you're no doubt stronger in body and mind.

I'm Athletic...
So are you...
We all are...

Vaughn Parker

Im Athletic 6 Month Workout Plan
Notes

No part of this book may be reproduced in any form or by any means without the prior written consent of the Publisher, excepting brief quotes used in reviews.

Book design, layout, and editing by Vaughn Parker

Disclaimer:
The author, publisher, and editor of this material are not responsible in any manner whatsoever for any injury that may occur through following the instructions contained in this material. The activities, physical and otherwise, described herein are for informational purposes only. They may be too strenuous or dangerous for some people and the reader(s) should consult a physician before engaging in this or any other fitness program.

Before you start...

Don't forget to warm up!

Check out the Dynamic Flow Drills page for one of 6 possible warm-ups. These drills are meant to flow from one exercise to the next without stopping, not even when the routine calls for you to switch hands. Repeat the warm-up between 2-5 times – or until you feel you are sufficiently warmed up.

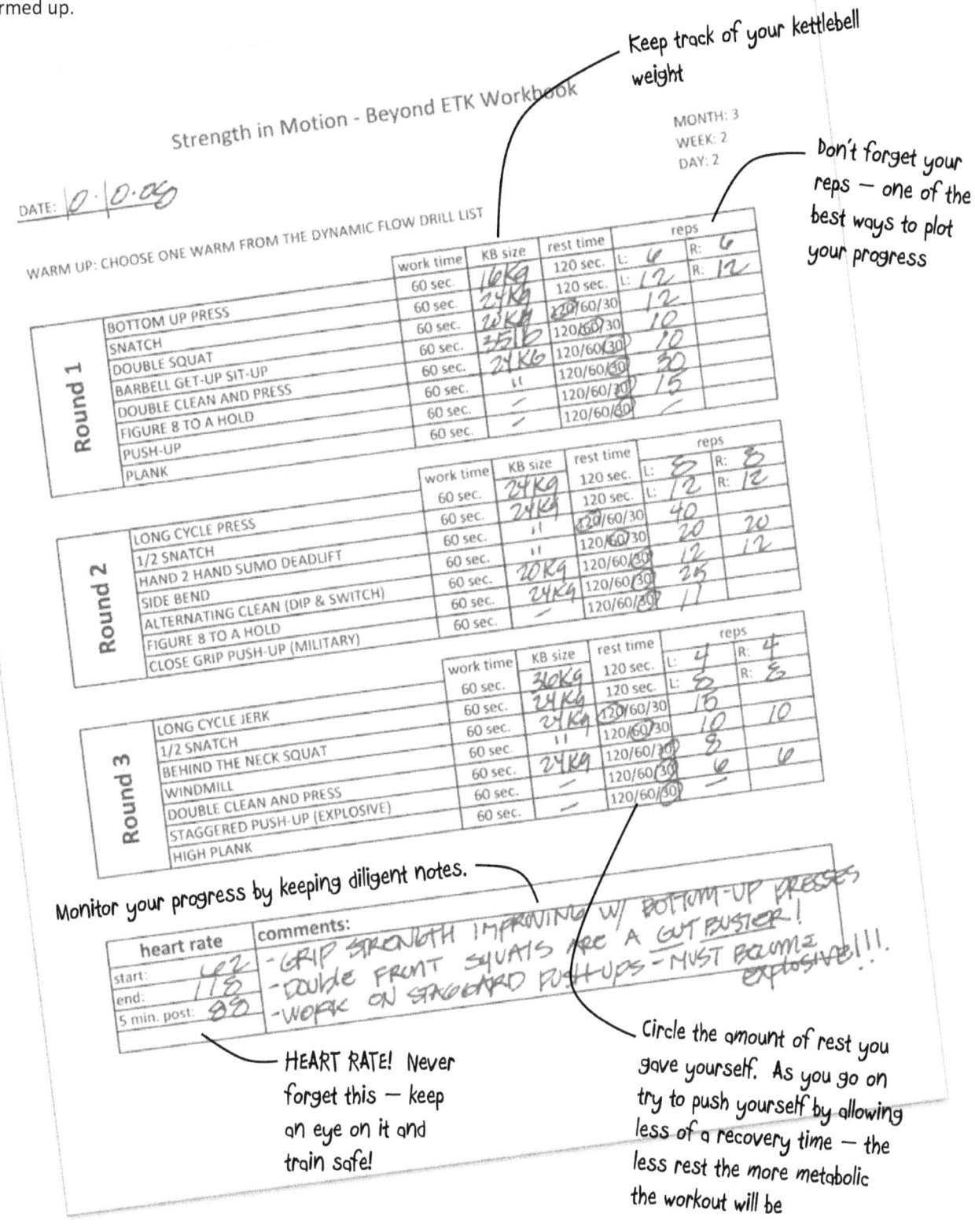

Keep track of your kettlebell weight

Don't forget your reps – one of the best ways to plot your progress

Monitor your progress by keeping diligent notes.

HEART RATE! Never forget this – keep an eye on it and train safe!

Circle the amount of rest you gave yourself. As you go on try to push yourself by allowing less of a recovery time – the less rest the more metabolic the workout will be

Get started

That's about it. The program you are starting may well prove more physically demanding than anything you've ever attempted. Make the commitment to complete all 4 weeks before you pick up that first kettlebell. Though the volume and work performed this week will certainly be easy compared to later weeks, it may be quite a shock to the system if you are just getting started with kettlebells.

Train safe…

Im Athletic 6 Month Workout Plan

Dynamic Flow Drill Warm-ups

DFD1	repeat 2-5x		DFD2	repeat 2-5x
	SWINGS x10			SWINGS 10-30 L,R
	CLEAN AND PRESS x5			SNATCH X1 L,R
	SQUAT (KB RACKED) x5			WINDMILL X1 L,R
	SNATCH x5			TGU X1 L,R

DFD3	repeat 2-5x		DFD4	repeat 2-5x
	SWINGS x3			SQUAT THRUST SNATCH L,R x6 (ALT.)
	SNATCH x3			SQUAT THRUST C&P L,R x6 (ALT.)
	OVERHEAD SQUAT x3			

DFD5	repeat 2-5x		DFD6	repeat 2-5x
	SQUAT & KICK (KB RACKED) x5 L,R			1 ARM SWING 30 sec. L,R
	BACK LUNGE TO PRESS x5 L,R			JUMP SQUAT 30 sec.
	FIGURE 8 TO HOLD x20 L,R			HALOS 30 sec. L,R

Im Athletic 6 Month Workout Plan

DATE: _____

WARM UP: CHOOSE ONE WARM FROM THE DYNAMIC FLOW DRILL LIST

		work time	KB size	rest time	reps	
Round 1	ONE ARM PRESS	30 sec.		60 sec.	L:	R:
	1/2 SNATCH	30 sec.		60 sec.	L:	R:
	DOUBLE SQUAT	30 sec.		60/30/15		
	BARBELL GET-UP SIT-UP	30 sec.		60/30/15		
	DOUBLE KB DEAD CLEAN	30 sec.		60/30/15		
	FIGURE 8 TO A HOLD	30 sec.		60/30/15		
	PUSH-UP	30 sec.		60/30/15		
	PLANK	30 sec.		60/30/15		

		work time	KB size	rest time	reps	
Round 2	ONE ARM PUSHPRESS	30 sec.		60 sec.	L:	R:
	SNATCH	30 sec.		60 sec.	L:	R:
	HAND 2 HAND SUMO DEADLIFT	30 sec.		60/30/15		
	SIDE BEND (LEFT AND RIGHT)	30 sec.		60/30/15		
	ALTERNATING CLEAN (DIP & SWITCH)	30 sec.		60/30/15		
	FIGURE 8 TO A HOLD	30 sec.		60/30/15		
	CLOSE GRIP PUSH-UP (MILITARY)	30 sec.		60/30/15		

		work time	KB size	rest time	reps	
Round 3	LONG CYCLE JERK	30 sec.		60 sec.	L:	R:
	1/2 SNATCH	30 sec.		60 sec.	L:	R:
	BEHIND THE NECK SQUAT	30 sec.		60/30/15		
	WINDMILL (LEFT AND RIGHT)	30 sec.		60/30/15		
	DOUBLE KB LONG CYCLE CLEAN	30 sec.		60/30/15		
	STAGGERED PUSH-UP (EXPLOSIVE)	30 sec.		60/30/15		
	HIGH PLANK	30 sec.		60/30/15		

heart rate	comments:
start:	
end:	
5 min. post:	

Im Athletic 6 Month Workout Plan

DATE: _____

WARM UP: CHOOSE ONE WARM FROM THE DYNAMIC FLOW DRILL LIST

		work time	KB size	rest time	reps	
Round 1	ONE ARM PRESS	30 sec.		60 sec.	L:	R:
	1/2 SNATCH	30 sec.		60 sec.	L:	R:
	DOUBLE SQUAT	30 sec.		60/30/15		
	BARBELL GET-UP SIT-UP	30 sec.		60/30/15		
	DOUBLE KB DEAD CLEAN	30 sec.		60/30/15		
	FIGURE 8 TO A HOLD	30 sec.		60/30/15		
	PUSH-UP	30 sec.		60/30/15		
	PLANK	30 sec.		60/30/15		

		work time	KB size	rest time	reps	
Round 2	ONE ARM PUSHPRESS	30 sec.		60 sec.	L:	R:
	SNATCH	30 sec.		60 sec.	L:	R:
	HAND 2 HAND SUMO DEADLIFT	30 sec.		60/30/15		
	SIDE BEND (LEFT AND RIGHT)	30 sec.		60/30/15		
	ALTERNATING CLEAN (DIP & SWITCH)	30 sec.		60/30/15		
	FIGURE 8 TO A HOLD	30 sec.		60/30/15		
	CLOSE GRIP PUSH-UP (MILITARY)	30 sec.		60/30/15		

		work time	KB size	rest time	reps	
Round 3	LONG CYCLE JERK	30 sec.		60 sec.	L:	R:
	1/2 SNATCH	30 sec.		60 sec.	L:	R:
	BEHIND THE NECK SQUAT	30 sec.		60/30/15		
	WINDMILL (LEFT AND RIGHT)	30 sec.		60/30/15		
	DOUBLE KB LONG CYCLE CLEAN	30 sec.		60/30/15		
	STAGGERED PUSH-UP (EXPLOSIVE)	30 sec.		60/30/15		
	HIGH PLANK	30 sec.		60/30/15		

heart rate	comments:
start:	
end:	
5 min. post:	

Im Athletic 6 Month Workout Plan

DATE: _____

WARM UP: CHOOSE ONE WARM FROM THE DYNAMIC FLOW DRILL LIST

		work time	KB size	rest time	reps	
Round 1	ONE ARM PRESS	30 sec.		60 sec.	L:	R:
	1/2 SNATCH	30 sec.		60 sec.	L:	R:
	DOUBLE SQUAT	30 sec.		60/30/15		
	BARBELL GET-UP SIT-UP	30 sec.		60/30/15		
	DOUBLE KB DEAD CLEAN	30 sec.		60/30/15		
	FIGURE 8 TO A HOLD	30 sec.		60/30/15		
	PUSH-UP	30 sec.		60/30/15		
	PLANK	30 sec.		60/30/15		

		work time	KB size	rest time	reps	
Round 2	ONE ARM PUSHPRESS	30 sec.		60 sec.	L:	R:
	SNATCH	30 sec.		60 sec.	L:	R:
	HAND 2 HAND SUMO DEADLIFT	30 sec.		60/30/15		
	SIDE BEND (LEFT AND RIGHT)	30 sec.		60/30/15		
	ALTERNATING CLEAN (DIP & SWITCH)	30 sec.		60/30/15		
	FIGURE 8 TO A HOLD	30 sec.		60/30/15		
	CLOSE GRIP PUSH-UP (MILITARY)	30 sec.		60/30/15		

		work time	KB size	rest time	reps	
Round 3	LONG CYCLE JERK	30 sec.		60 sec.	L:	R:
	1/2 SNATCH	30 sec.		60 sec.	L:	R:
	BEHIND THE NECK SQUAT	30 sec.		60/30/15		
	WINDMILL (LEFT AND RIGHT)	30 sec.		60/30/15		
	DOUBLE KB LONG CYCLE CLEAN	30 sec.		60/30/15		
	STAGGERED PUSH-UP (EXPLOSIVE)	30 sec.		60/30/15		
	HIGH PLANK	30 sec.		60/30/15		

heart rate	comments:
start:	
end:	
5 min. post:	

Im Athletic 6 Month Workout Plan

DATE: _____

WARM UP: CHOOSE ONE WARM FROM THE DYNAMIC FLOW DRILL LIST

		work time	KB size	rest time	reps	
Round 1	ONE ARM PRESS	30 sec.		60 sec.	L:	R:
	1/2 SNATCH	30 sec.		60 sec.	L:	R:
	DOUBLE SQUAT	30 sec.		60/30/15		
	BARBELL GET-UP SIT-UP	30 sec.		60/30/15		
	DOUBLE KB DEAD CLEAN	30 sec.		60/30/15		
	FIGURE 8 TO A HOLD	30 sec.		60/30/15		
	PUSH-UP	30 sec.		60/30/15		
	PLANK	30 sec.		60/30/15		

		work time	KB size	rest time	reps	
Round 2	ONE ARM PUSHPRESS	30 sec.		60 sec.	L:	R:
	SNATCH	30 sec.		60 sec.	L:	R:
	HAND 2 HAND SUMO DEADLIFT	30 sec.		60/30/15		
	SIDE BEND (LEFT AND RIGHT)	30 sec.		60/30/15		
	ALTERNATING CLEAN (DIP & SWITCH)	30 sec.		60/30/15		
	FIGURE 8 TO A HOLD	30 sec.		60/30/15		
	CLOSE GRIP PUSH-UP (MILITARY)	30 sec.		60/30/15		

		work time	KB size	rest time	reps	
Round 3	LONG CYCLE JERK	30 sec.		60 sec.	L:	R:
	1/2 SNATCH	30 sec.		60 sec.	L:	R:
	BEHIND THE NECK SQUAT	30 sec.		60/30/15		
	WINDMILL (LEFT AND RIGHT)	30 sec.		60/30/15		
	DOUBLE KB LONG CYCLE CLEAN	30 sec.		60/30/15		
	STAGGERED PUSH-UP (EXPLOSIVE)	30 sec.		60/30/15		
	HIGH PLANK	30 sec.		60/30/15		

heart rate	comments:
start:	
end:	
5 min. post:	

Im Athletic 6 Month Workout Plan

DATE: _____

WARM UP: CHOOSE ONE WARM FROM THE DYNAMIC FLOW DRILL LIST

		work time	KB size	rest time	reps	
Round 1	BOTTOM UP PRESS	30 sec.		45 sec.	L:	R:
	SNATCH	30 sec.		45 sec.	L:	R:
	DOUBLE SQUAT	30 sec.		60/30/15		
	BARBELL GET-UP SIT-UP	30 sec.		60/30/15		
	DOUBLE KB DEAD CLEAN	30 sec.		60/30/15		
	FIGURE 8 TO A HOLD	30 sec.		60/30/15		
	PUSH-UP	30 sec.		60/30/15		
	PLANK	30 sec.		60/30/15		

		work time	KB size	rest time	reps	
Round 2	LONG CYCLE PRESS	30 sec.		45 sec.	L:	R:
	1/2 SNATCH	30 sec.		45 sec.	L:	R:
	HAND 2 HAND SUMO DEADLIFT	30 sec.		60/30/15		
	SIDE BEND (LEFT AND RIGHT)	30 sec.		60/30/15		
	ALTERNATING CLEAN (DIP & SWITCH)	30 sec.		60/30/15		
	FIGURE 8 TO A HOLD	30 sec.		60/30/15		
	CLOSE GRIP PUSH-UP (MILITARY)	30 sec.		60/30/15		

		work time	KB size	rest time	reps	
Round 3	JERK	30 sec.		45 sec.	L:	R:
	SNATCH	30 sec.		45 sec.	L:	R:
	BEHIND THE NECK SQUAT	30 sec.		60/30/15		
	WINDMILL (LEFT AND RIGHT)	30 sec.		60/30/15		
	DOUBLE KB LONG CYCLE CLEAN	30 sec.		60/30/15		
	STAGGERED PUSH-UP (EXPLOSIVE)	30 sec.		60/30/15		
	HIGH PLANK	30 sec.		60/30/15		

heart rate	comments:
start:	
end:	
5 min. post:	

Im Athletic 6 Month Workout Plan

WARM UP: CHOOSE ONE WARM FROM THE DYNAMIC FLOW DRILL LIST

		work time	KB size	rest time	reps		
Round 1	BOTTOM UP PRESS	30 sec.		45 sec.	L:		R:
	SNATCH	30 sec.		45 sec.	L:		R:
	DOUBLE SQUAT	30 sec.		60/30/15			
	BARBELL GET-UP SIT-UP	30 sec.		60/30/15			
	DOUBLE KB DEAD CLEAN	30 sec.		60/30/15			
	FIGURE 8 TO A HOLD	30 sec.		60/30/15			
	PUSH-UP	30 sec.		60/30/15			
	PLANK	30 sec.		60/30/15			

		work time	KB size	rest time	reps		
Round 2	LONG CYCLE PRESS	30 sec.		45 sec.	L:		R:
	1/2 SNATCH	30 sec.		45 sec.	L:		R:
	HAND 2 HAND SUMO DEADLIFT	30 sec.		60/30/15			
	SIDE BEND (LEFT AND RIGHT)	30 sec.		60/30/15			
	ALTERNATING CLEAN (DIP & SWITCH)	30 sec.		60/30/15			
	FIGURE 8 TO A HOLD	30 sec.		60/30/15			
	CLOSE GRIP PUSH-UP (MILITARY)	30 sec.		60/30/15			

		work time	KB size	rest time	reps		
Round 3	JERK	30 sec.		45 sec.	L:		R:
	SNATCH	30 sec.		45 sec.	L:		R:
	BEHIND THE NECK SQUAT	30 sec.		60/30/15			
	WINDMILL (LEFT AND RIGHT)	30 sec.		60/30/15			
	DOUBLE KB LONG CYCLE CLEAN	30 sec.		60/30/15			
	STAGGERED PUSH-UP (EXPLOSIVE)	30 sec.		60/30/15			
	HIGH PLANK	30 sec.		60/30/15			

heart rate	comments:
start:	
end:	
5 min. post:	

Im Athletic 6 Month Workout Plan

DATE: _____

WARM UP: CHOOSE ONE WARM FROM THE DYNAMIC FLOW DRILL LIST

		work time	KB size	rest time	reps	
Round 1	BOTTOM UP PRESS	30 sec.		45 sec.	L:	R:
	SNATCH	30 sec.		45 sec.	L:	R:
	DOUBLE SQUAT	30 sec.		60/30/15		
	BARBELL GET-UP SIT-UP	30 sec.		60/30/15		
	DOUBLE KB DEAD CLEAN	30 sec.		60/30/15		
	FIGURE 8 TO A HOLD	30 sec.		60/30/15		
	PUSH-UP	30 sec.		60/30/15		
	PLANK	30 sec.		60/30/15		

		work time	KB size	rest time	reps	
Round 2	LONG CYCLE PRESS	30 sec.		45 sec.	L:	R:
	1/2 SNATCH	30 sec.		45 sec.	L:	R:
	HAND 2 HAND SUMO DEADLIFT	30 sec.		60/30/15		
	SIDE BEND (LEFT AND RIGHT)	30 sec.		60/30/15		
	ALTERNATING CLEAN (DIP & SWITCH)	30 sec.		60/30/15		
	FIGURE 8 TO A HOLD	30 sec.		60/30/15		
	CLOSE GRIP PUSH-UP (MILITARY)	30 sec.		60/30/15		

		work time	KB size	rest time	reps	
Round 3	JERK	30 sec.		45 sec.	L:	R:
	SNATCH	30 sec.		45 sec.	L:	R:
	BEHIND THE NECK SQUAT	30 sec.		60/30/15		
	WINDMILL (LEFT AND RIGHT)	30 sec.		60/30/15		
	DOUBLE KB LONG CYCLE CLEAN	30 sec.		60/30/15		
	STAGGERED PUSH-UP (EXPLOSIVE)	30 sec.		60/30/15		
	HIGH PLANK	30 sec.		60/30/15		

heart rate	comments:
start:	
end:	
5 min. post:	

Im Athletic 6 Month Workout Plan

DATE: _____

WARM UP: CHOOSE ONE WARM FROM THE DYNAMIC FLOW DRILL LIST

		work time	KB size	rest time	reps	
Round 1	BOTTOM UP PRESS	30 sec.		30 sec.	L:	R:
	SNATCH	30 sec.		30 sec.	L:	R:
	DOUBLE SQUAT	30 sec.		60/30/15		
	BARBELL GET-UP SIT-UP	30 sec.		60/30/15		
	DOUBLE KB DEAD CLEAN	30 sec.		60/30/15		
	FIGURE 8 TO A HOLD	30 sec.		60/30/15		
	PUSH-UP	30 sec.		60/30/15		
	PLANK	30 sec.		60/30/15		

		work time	KB size	rest time	reps	
Round 2	LONG CYCLE PRESS	30 sec.		30 sec.	L:	R:
	1/2 SNATCH	30 sec.		30 sec.	L:	R:
	HAND 2 HAND SUMO DEADLIFT	30 sec.		60/30/15		
	SIDE BEND (LEFT AND RIGHT)	30 sec.		60/30/15		
	ALTERNATING CLEAN (DIP & SWITCH)	30 sec.		60/30/15		
	FIGURE 8 TO A HOLD	30 sec.		60/30/15		
	CLOSE GRIP PUSH-UP (MILITARY)	30 sec.		60/30/15		

		work time	KB size	rest time	reps	
Round 3	JERK	30 sec.		30 sec.	L:	R:
	SNATCH	30 sec.		30 sec.	L:	R:
	BEHIND THE NECK SQUAT	30 sec.		60/30/15		
	WINDMILL (LEFT AND RIGHT)	30 sec.		60/30/15		
	DOUBLE KB LONG CYCLE CLEAN	30 sec.		60/30/15		
	STAGGERED PUSH-UP (EXPLOSIVE)	30 sec.		60/30/15		
	HIGH PLANK	30 sec.		60/30/15		

heart rate	comments:
start:	
end:	
5 min. post:	

Im Athletic 6 Month Workout Plan

DATE: _____

WARM UP: CHOOSE ONE WARM FROM THE DYNAMIC FLOW DRILL LIST

		work time	KB size	rest time	reps	
Round 1	LONG CYCLE JERK	30 sec.		30 sec.	L:	R:
	1/2 SNATCH	30 sec.		30 sec.	L:	R:
	DOUBLE SQUAT	30 sec.		60/30/15		
	BARBELL GET-UP SIT-UP	30 sec.		60/30/15		
	DOUBLE KB DEAD CLEAN	30 sec.		60/30/15		
	FIGURE 8 TO A HOLD	30 sec.		60/30/15		
	PUSH-UP	30 sec.		60/30/15		
	PLANK	30 sec.		60/30/15		

		work time	KB size	rest time	reps	
Round 2	JERK	30 sec.		30 sec.	L:	R:
	SNATCH	30 sec.		30 sec.	L:	R:
	HAND 2 HAND SUMO DEADLIFT	30 sec.		60/30/15		
	SIDE BEND (LEFT AND RIGHT)	30 sec.		60/30/15		
	ALTERNATING CLEAN (DIP & SWITCH)	30 sec.		60/30/15		
	FIGURE 8 TO A HOLD	30 sec.		60/30/15		
	CLOSE GRIP PUSH-UP (MILITARY)	30 sec.		60/30/15		

		work time	KB size	rest time	reps	
Round 3	BOTTOM UP PUSH PRESS	30 sec.		30 sec.	L:	R:
	1/2 SNATCH	30 sec.		30 sec.	L:	R:
	BEHIND THE NECK SQUAT	30 sec.		60/30/15		
	WINDMILL (LEFT AND RIGHT)	30 sec.		60/30/15		
	DOUBLE KB LONG CYCLE CLEAN	30 sec.		60/30/15		
	STAGGERED PUSH-UP (EXPLOSIVE)	30 sec.		60/30/15		
	HIGH PLANK	30 sec.		60/30/15		

heart rate	comments:
start:	
end:	
5 min. post:	

Im Athletic 6 Month Workout Plan

WARM UP: CHOOSE ONE WARM FROM THE DYNAMIC FLOW DRILL LIST

		work time	KB size	rest time	reps	
Round 1	LONG CYCLE JERK	30 sec.		30 sec.	L:	R:
	1/2 SNATCH	30 sec.		30 sec.	L:	R:
	DOUBLE SQUAT	30 sec.		60/30/15		
	BARBELL GET-UP SIT-UP	30 sec.		60/30/15		
	DOUBLE KB DEAD CLEAN	30 sec.		60/30/15		
	FIGURE 8 TO A HOLD	30 sec.		60/30/15		
	PUSH-UP	30 sec.		60/30/15		
	PLANK	30 sec.		60/30/15		

		work time	KB size	rest time	reps	
Round 2	JERK	30 sec.		30 sec.	L:	R:
	SNATCH	30 sec.		30 sec.	L:	R:
	HAND 2 HAND SUMO DEADLIFT	30 sec.		60/30/15		
	SIDE BEND (LEFT AND RIGHT)	30 sec.		60/30/15		
	ALTERNATING CLEAN (DIP & SWITCH)	30 sec.		60/30/15		
	FIGURE 8 TO A HOLD	30 sec.		60/30/15		
	CLOSE GRIP PUSH-UP (MILITARY)	30 sec.		60/30/15		

		work time	KB size	rest time	reps	
Round 3	BOTTOM UP PUSH PRESS	30 sec.		30 sec.	L:	R:
	1/2 SNATCH	30 sec.		30 sec.	L:	R:
	BEHIND THE NECK SQUAT	30 sec.		60/30/15		
	WINDMILL (LEFT AND RIGHT)	30 sec.		60/30/15		
	DOUBLE KB LONG CYCLE CLEAN	30 sec.		60/30/15		
	STAGGERED PUSH-UP (EXPLOSIVE)	30 sec.		60/30/15		
	HIGH PLANK	30 sec.		60/30/15		

heart rate	comments:
start:	
end:	
5 min. post:	

Im Athletic 6 Month Workout Plan

DATE: _____

WARM UP: CHOOSE ONE WARM FROM THE DYNAMIC FLOW DRILL LIST

Round 1		work time	KB size	rest time	reps	
	LONG CYCLE JERK	30 sec.		30 sec.	L:	R:
	1/2 SNATCH	30 sec.		30 sec.	L:	R:
	DOUBLE SQUAT	30 sec.		60/30/15		
	BARBELL GET-UP SIT-UP	30 sec.		60/30/15		
	DOUBLE KB DEAD CLEAN	30 sec.		60/30/15		
	FIGURE 8 TO A HOLD	30 sec.		60/30/15		
	PUSH-UP	30 sec.		60/30/15		
	PLANK	30 sec.		60/30/15		

Round 2		work time	KB size	rest time	reps	
	JERK	30 sec.		30 sec.	L:	R:
	SNATCH	30 sec.		30 sec.	L:	R:
	HAND 2 HAND SUMO DEADLIFT	30 sec.		60/30/15		
	SIDE BEND (LEFT AND RIGHT)	30 sec.		60/30/15		
	ALTERNATING CLEAN (DIP & SWITCH)	30 sec.		60/30/15		
	FIGURE 8 TO A HOLD	30 sec.		60/30/15		
	CLOSE GRIP PUSH-UP (MILITARY)	30 sec.		60/30/15		

Round 3		work time	KB size	rest time	reps	
	BOTTOM UP PUSH PRESS	30 sec.		30 sec.	L:	R:
	1/2 SNATCH	30 sec.		30 sec.	L:	R:
	BEHIND THE NECK SQUAT	30 sec.		60/30/15		
	WINDMILL (LEFT AND RIGHT)	30 sec.		60/30/15		
	DOUBLE KB LONG CYCLE CLEAN	30 sec.		60/30/15		
	STAGGERED PUSH-UP (EXPLOSIVE)	30 sec.		60/30/15		
	HIGH PLANK	30 sec.		60/30/15		

heart rate	comments:
start:	
end:	
5 min. post:	

Im Athletic 6 Month Workout Plan

DATE: _____

WARM UP: CHOOSE ONE WARM FROM THE DYNAMIC FLOW DRILL LIST

		work time	KB size	rest time	reps	
Round 1	LONG CYCLE JERK	30 sec.		30 sec.	L:	R:
	1/2 SNATCH	30 sec.		30 sec.	L:	R:
	DOUBLE SQUAT	30 sec.		60/30/15		
	BARBELL GET-UP SIT-UP	30 sec.		60/30/15		
	DOUBLE KB DEAD CLEAN	30 sec.		60/30/15		
	FIGURE 8 TO A HOLD	30 sec.		60/30/15		
	PUSH-UP	30 sec.		60/30/15		
	PLANK	30 sec.		60/30/15		

		work time	KB size	rest time	reps	
Round 2	JERK	30 sec.		30 sec.	L:	R:
	SNATCH	30 sec.		30 sec.	L:	R:
	HAND 2 HAND SUMO DEADLIFT	30 sec.		60/30/15		
	SIDE BEND (LEFT AND RIGHT)	30 sec.		60/30/15		
	ALTERNATING CLEAN (DIP & SWITCH)	30 sec.		60/30/15		
	FIGURE 8 TO A HOLD	30 sec.		60/30/15		
	CLOSE GRIP PUSH-UP (MILITARY)	30 sec.		60/30/15		

		work time	KB size	rest time	reps	
Round 3	BOTTOM UP PUSH PRESS	30 sec.		30 sec.	L:	R:
	1/2 SNATCH	30 sec.		30 sec.	L:	R:
	BEHIND THE NECK SQUAT	30 sec.		60/30/15		
	WINDMILL (LEFT AND RIGHT)	30 sec.		60/30/15		
	DOUBLE KB LONG CYCLE CLEAN	30 sec.		60/30/15		
	STAGGERED PUSH-UP (EXPLOSIVE)	30 sec.		60/30/15		
	HIGH PLANK	30 sec.		60/30/15		

heart rate	comments:
start:	
end:	
5 min. post:	

Im Athletic 6 Month Workout Plan

DATE: _____

WARM UP: CHOOSE ONE WARM FROM THE DYNAMIC FLOW DRILL LIST

		work time	KB size	rest time	reps	
Round 1	PRESS	30 sec.		15 sec.	L:	R:
	SNATCH	30 sec.		15 sec.	L:	R:
	DOUBLE SQUAT	30 sec.		60/30/15		
	BARBELL GET-UP SIT-UP	30 sec.		60/30/15		
	DOUBLE KB DEAD CLEAN	30 sec.		60/30/15		
	FIGURE 8 TO A HOLD	30 sec.		60/30/15		
	PUSH-UP	30 sec.		60/30/15		
	PLANK	30 sec.		60/30/15		

		work time	KB size	rest time	reps	
Round 2	LONG CYCLE JERK	30 sec.		15 sec.	L:	R:
	SNATCH	30 sec.		15 sec.	L:	R:
	HAND 2 HAND SUMO DEADLIFT	30 sec.		60/30/15		
	SIDE BEND (LEFT AND RIGHT)	30 sec.		60/30/15		
	ALTERNATING CLEAN (DIP & SWITCH)	30 sec.		60/30/15		
	FIGURE 8 TO A HOLD	30 sec.		60/30/15		
	CLOSE GRIP PUSH-UP (MILITARY)	30 sec.		60/30/15		

		work time	KB size	rest time	reps	
Round 3	JERK	30 sec.		15 sec.	L:	R:
	1/2 SNATCH	30 sec.		15 sec.	L:	R:
	BEHIND THE NECK SQUAT	30 sec.		60/30/15		
	WINDMILL (LEFT AND RIGHT)	30 sec.		60/30/15		
	DOUBLE KB LONG CYCLE CLEAN	30 sec.		60/30/15		
	STAGGERED PUSH-UP (EXPLOSIVE)	30 sec.		60/30/15		
	HIGH PLANK	30 sec.		60/30/15		

heart rate	comments:
start:	
end:	
5 min. post:	

Im Athletic 6 Month Workout Plan

DATE: _____

WARM UP: CHOOSE ONE WARM FROM THE DYNAMIC FLOW DRILL LIST

		work time	KB size	rest time	reps	
Round 1	PRESS	30 sec.		15 sec.	L:	R:
	SNATCH	30 sec.		15 sec.	L:	R:
	DOUBLE SQUAT	30 sec.		60/30/15		
	BARBELL GET-UP SIT-UP	30 sec.		60/30/15		
	DOUBLE KB DEAD CLEAN	30 sec.		60/30/15		
	FIGURE 8 TO A HOLD	30 sec.		60/30/15		
	PUSH-UP	30 sec.		60/30/15		
	PLANK	30 sec.		60/30/15		

		work time	KB size	rest time	reps	
Round 2	LONG CYCLE JERK	30 sec.		15 sec.	L:	R:
	SNATCH	30 sec.		15 sec.	L:	R:
	HAND 2 HAND SUMO DEADLIFT	30 sec.		60/30/15		
	SIDE BEND (LEFT AND RIGHT)	30 sec.		60/30/15		
	ALTERNATING CLEAN (DIP & SWITCH)	30 sec.		60/30/15		
	FIGURE 8 TO A HOLD	30 sec.		60/30/15		
	CLOSE GRIP PUSH-UP (MILITARY)	30 sec.		60/30/15		

		work time	KB size	rest time	reps	
Round 3	JERK	30 sec.		15 sec.	L:	R:
	1/2 SNATCH	30 sec.		15 sec.	L:	R:
	BEHIND THE NECK SQUAT	30 sec.		60/30/15		
	WINDMILL (LEFT AND RIGHT)	30 sec.		60/30/15		
	DOUBLE KB LONG CYCLE CLEAN	30 sec.		60/30/15		
	STAGGERED PUSH-UP (EXPLOSIVE)	30 sec.		60/30/15		
	HIGH PLANK	30 sec.		60/30/15		

heart rate	comments:
start:	
end:	
5 min. post:	

Im Athletic 6 Month Workout Plan

DATE: _____

MONTH: 1
WEEK: 4
DAY: 3

WARM UP: CHOOSE ONE WARM FROM THE DYNAMIC FLOW DRILL LIST

		work time	KB size	rest time	reps	
Round 1	PRESS	30 sec.		15 sec.	L:	R:
	SNATCH	30 sec.		15 sec.	L:	R:
	DOUBLE SQUAT	30 sec.		60/30/15		
	BARBELL GET-UP SIT-UP	30 sec.		60/30/15		
	DOUBLE KB DEAD CLEAN	30 sec.		60/30/15		
	FIGURE 8 TO A HOLD	30 sec.		60/30/15		
	PUSH-UP	30 sec.		60/30/15		
	PLANK	30 sec.		60/30/15		

		work time	KB size	rest time	reps	
Round 2	LONG CYCLE JERK	30 sec.		15 sec.	L:	R:
	SNATCH	30 sec.		15 sec.	L:	R:
	HAND 2 HAND SUMO DEADLIFT	30 sec.		60/30/15		
	SIDE BEND (LEFT AND RIGHT)	30 sec.		60/30/15		
	ALTERNATING CLEAN (DIP & SWITCH)	30 sec.		60/30/15		
	FIGURE 8 TO A HOLD	30 sec.		60/30/15		
	CLOSE GRIP PUSH-UP (MILITARY)	30 sec.		60/30/15		

		work time	KB size	rest time	reps	
Round 3	JERK	30 sec.		15 sec.	L:	R:
	1/2 SNATCH	30 sec.		15 sec.	L:	R:
	BEHIND THE NECK SQUAT	30 sec.		60/30/15		
	WINDMILL (LEFT AND RIGHT)	30 sec.		60/30/15		
	DOUBLE KB LONG CYCLE CLEAN	30 sec.		60/30/15		
	STAGGERED PUSH-UP (EXPLOSIVE)	30 sec.		60/30/15		
	HIGH PLANK	30 sec.		60/30/15		

heart rate	comments:
start:	
end:	
5 min. post:	

Im Athletic 6 Month Workout Plan

DATE: _____

WARM UP: CHOOSE ONE WARM FROM THE DYNAMIC FLOW DRILL LIST

Round 1		work time	KB size	rest time	reps	
	PRESS	30 sec.		15 sec.	L:	R:
	SNATCH	30 sec.		15 sec.	L:	R:
	DOUBLE SQUAT	30 sec.		60/30/15		
	BARBELL GET-UP SIT-UP	30 sec.		60/30/15		
	DOUBLE KB DEAD CLEAN	30 sec.		60/30/15		
	FIGURE 8 TO A HOLD	30 sec.		60/30/15		
	PUSH-UP	30 sec.		60/30/15		
	PLANK	30 sec.		60/30/15		

Round 2		work time	KB size	rest time	reps	
	LONG CYCLE JERK	30 sec.		15 sec.	L:	R:
	SNATCH	30 sec.		15 sec.	L:	R:
	HAND 2 HAND SUMO DEADLIFT	30 sec.		60/30/15		
	SIDE BEND (LEFT AND RIGHT)	30 sec.		60/30/15		
	ALTERNATING CLEAN (DIP & SWITCH)	30 sec.		60/30/15		
	FIGURE 8 TO A HOLD	30 sec.		60/30/15		
	CLOSE GRIP PUSH-UP (MILITARY)	30 sec.		60/30/15		

Round 3		work time	KB size	rest time	reps	
	JERK	30 sec.		15 sec.	L:	R:
	1/2 SNATCH	30 sec.		15 sec.	L:	R:
	BEHIND THE NECK SQUAT	30 sec.		60/30/15		
	WINDMILL (LEFT AND RIGHT)	30 sec.		60/30/15		
	DOUBLE KB LONG CYCLE CLEAN	30 sec.		60/30/15		
	STAGGERED PUSH-UP (EXPLOSIVE)	30 sec.		60/30/15		
	HIGH PLANK	30 sec.		60/30/15		

heart rate	comments:
start:	
end:	
5 min. post:	

You've finished month 1!

"Every day you have to test yourself. If you don't, it's a wasted day."
Terry Butts, Marine Corps

Im Athletic 6 Month Workout Plan

DATE: _____

WARM UP: CHOOSE ONE WARM FROM THE DYNAMIC FLOW DRILL LIST

Round 1		work time	KB size	rest time	reps	
	BOTTOM UP PRESS	45 sec.		90 sec.	L:	R:
	SNATCH	45 sec.		90 sec.	L:	R:
	DOUBLE SQUAT	30 sec.		60/30/15		
	BARBELL GET-UP SIT-UP	30 sec.		60/30/15		
	DOUBLE KB DEAD CLEAN	30 sec.		60/30/15		
	FIGURE 8 TO A HOLD	30 sec.		60/30/15		
	PUSH-UP	30 sec.		60/30/15		
	PLANK	30 sec.		60/30/15		

Round 2		work time	KB size	rest time	reps	
	ONE ARM JERK	45 sec.		90 sec.	L:	R:
	1/2 SNATCH	45 sec.		90 sec.	L:	R:
	HAND 2 HAND SUMO DEADLIFT	30 sec.		60/30/15		
	SIDE BEND (LEFT AND RIGHT)	30 sec.		60/30/15		
	ALTERNATING CLEAN (DIP & SWITCH)	30 sec.		60/30/15		
	FIGURE 8 TO A HOLD	30 sec.		60/30/15		
	CLOSE GRIP PUSH-UP (MILITARY)	30 sec.		60/30/15		

Round 3		work time	KB size	rest time	reps	
	LONG CYCLE BOTTOM UP JERK	45 sec.		90 sec.	L:	R:
	1/2 SNATCH	45 sec.		90 sec.	L:	R:
	BEHIND THE NECK SQUAT	30 sec.		60/30/15		
	WINDMILL (LEFT AND RIGHT)	30 sec.		60/30/15		
	DOUBLE KB LONG CYCLE CLEAN	30 sec.		60/30/15		
	STAGGERED PUSH-UP (EXPLOSIVE)	30 sec.		60/30/15		
	HIGH PLANK	30 sec.		60/30/15		

heart rate	comments:
start:	
end:	
5 min. post:	

Im Athletic 6 Month Workout Plan

DATE: _____

WARM UP: CHOOSE ONE WARM FROM THE DYNAMIC FLOW DRILL LIST

		work time	KB size	rest time	reps	
Round 1	BOTTOM UP PRESS	45 sec.		90 sec.	L:	R:
	SNATCH	45 sec.		90 sec.	L:	R:
	DOUBLE SQUAT	30 sec.		60/30/15		
	BARBELL GET-UP SIT-UP	30 sec.		60/30/15		
	DOUBLE KB DEAD CLEAN	30 sec.		60/30/15		
	FIGURE 8 TO A HOLD	30 sec.		60/30/15		
	PUSH-UP	30 sec.		60/30/15		
	PLANK	30 sec.		60/30/15		

		work time	KB size	rest time	reps	
Round 2	ONE ARM JERK	45 sec.		90 sec.	L:	R:
	1/2 SNATCH	45 sec.		90 sec.	L:	R:
	HAND 2 HAND SUMO DEADLIFT	30 sec.		60/30/15		
	SIDE BEND (LEFT AND RIGHT)	30 sec.		60/30/15		
	ALTERNATING CLEAN (DIP & SWITCH)	30 sec.		60/30/15		
	FIGURE 8 TO A HOLD	30 sec.		60/30/15		
	CLOSE GRIP PUSH-UP (MILITARY)	30 sec.		60/30/15		

		work time	KB size	rest time	reps	
Round 3	LONG CYCLE BOTTOM UP JERK	45 sec.		90 sec.	L:	R:
	1/2 SNATCH	45 sec.		90 sec.	L:	R:
	BEHIND THE NECK SQUAT	30 sec.		60/30/15		
	WINDMILL (LEFT AND RIGHT)	30 sec.		60/30/15		
	DOUBLE KB LONG CYCLE CLEAN	30 sec.		60/30/15		
	STAGGERED PUSH-UP (EXPLOSIVE)	30 sec.		60/30/15		
	HIGH PLANK	30 sec.		60/30/15		

heart rate	comments:
start:	
end:	
5 min. post:	

Im Athletic 6 Month Workout Plan

DATE: _____

WARM UP: CHOOSE ONE WARM FROM THE DYNAMIC FLOW DRILL LIST

		work time	KB size	rest time	reps	
Round 1	BOTTOM UP PRESS	45 sec.		90 sec.	L:	R:
	SNATCH	45 sec.		90 sec.	L:	R:
	DOUBLE SQUAT	30 sec.		60/30/15		
	BARBELL GET-UP SIT-UP	30 sec.		60/30/15		
	DOUBLE KB DEAD CLEAN	30 sec.		60/30/15		
	FIGURE 8 TO A HOLD	30 sec.		60/30/15		
	PUSH-UP	30 sec.		60/30/15		
	PLANK	30 sec.		60/30/15		

		work time	KB size	rest time	reps	
Round 2	ONE ARM JERK	45 sec.		90 sec.	L:	R:
	1/2 SNATCH	45 sec.		90 sec.	L:	R:
	HAND 2 HAND SUMO DEADLIFT	30 sec.		60/30/15		
	SIDE BEND (LEFT AND RIGHT)	30 sec.		60/30/15		
	ALTERNATING CLEAN (DIP & SWITCH)	30 sec.		60/30/15		
	FIGURE 8 TO A HOLD	30 sec.		60/30/15		
	CLOSE GRIP PUSH-UP (MILITARY)	30 sec.		60/30/15		

		work time	KB size	rest time	reps	
Round 3	LONG CYCLE BOTTOM UP JERK	45 sec.		90 sec.	L:	R:
	1/2 SNATCH	45 sec.		90 sec.	L:	R:
	BEHIND THE NECK SQUAT	30 sec.		60/30/15		
	WINDMILL (LEFT AND RIGHT)	30 sec.		60/30/15		
	DOUBLE KB LONG CYCLE CLEAN	30 sec.		60/30/15		
	STAGGERED PUSH-UP (EXPLOSIVE)	30 sec.		60/30/15		
	HIGH PLANK	30 sec.		60/30/15		

heart rate	comments:
start:	
end:	
5 min. post:	

Im Athletic 6 Month Workout Plan

DATE: _____

WARM UP: CHOOSE ONE WARM FROM THE DYNAMIC FLOW DRILL LIST

		work time	KB size	rest time	reps	
Round 1	BOTTOM UP PRESS	45 sec.		90 sec.	L:	R:
	SNATCH	45 sec.		90 sec.	L:	R:
	DOUBLE SQUAT	30 sec.		60/30/15		
	BARBELL GET-UP SIT-UP	30 sec.		60/30/15		
	DOUBLE KB DEAD CLEAN	30 sec.		60/30/15		
	FIGURE 8 TO A HOLD	30 sec.		60/30/15		
	PUSH-UP	30 sec.		60/30/15		
	PLANK	30 sec.		60/30/15		

		work time	KB size	rest time	reps	
Round 2	ONE ARM JERK	45 sec.		90 sec.	L:	R:
	1/2 SNATCH	45 sec.		90 sec.	L:	R:
	HAND 2 HAND SUMO DEADLIFT	30 sec.		60/30/15		
	SIDE BEND (LEFT AND RIGHT)	30 sec.		60/30/15		
	ALTERNATING CLEAN (DIP & SWITCH)	30 sec.		60/30/15		
	FIGURE 8 TO A HOLD	30 sec.		60/30/15		
	CLOSE GRIP PUSH-UP (MILITARY)	30 sec.		60/30/15		

		work time	KB size	rest time	reps	
Round 3	LONG CYCLE BOTTOM UP JERK	45 sec.		90 sec.	L:	R:
	1/2 SNATCH	45 sec.		90 sec.	L:	R:
	BEHIND THE NECK SQUAT	30 sec.		60/30/15		
	WINDMILL (LEFT AND RIGHT)	30 sec.		60/30/15		
	DOUBLE KB LONG CYCLE CLEAN	30 sec.		60/30/15		
	STAGGERED PUSH-UP (EXPLOSIVE)	30 sec.		60/30/15		
	HIGH PLANK	30 sec.		60/30/15		

heart rate	comments:
start:	
end:	
5 min. post:	

Im Athletic 6 Month Workout Plan

DATE: _____

WARM UP: CHOOSE ONE WARM FROM THE DYNAMIC FLOW DRILL LIST

		work time	KB size	rest time	reps	
Round 1	LONG CYCLE BOTTOM UP JERK	45 sec.		60 sec.	L:	R:
	SNATCH	45 sec.		60 sec.	L:	R:
	DOUBLE SQUAT	30 sec.		60/30/15		
	BARBELL GET-UP SIT-UP	30 sec.		60/30/15		
	DOUBLE KB DEAD CLEAN	30 sec.		60/30/15		
	FIGURE 8 TO A HOLD	30 sec.		60/30/15		
	PUSH-UP	30 sec.		60/30/15		
	PLANK	30 sec.		60/30/15		

		work time	KB size	rest time	reps	
Round 2	PRESS	45 sec.		60 sec.	L:	R:
	SNATCH	45 sec.		60 sec.	L:	R:
	HAND 2 HAND SUMO DEADLIFT	30 sec.		60/30/15		
	SIDE BEND (LEFT AND RIGHT)	30 sec.		60/30/15		
	ALTERNATING CLEAN (DIP & SWITCH)	30 sec.		60/30/15		
	FIGURE 8 TO A HOLD	30 sec.		60/30/15		
	CLOSE GRIP PUSH-UP (MILITARY)	30 sec.		60/30/15		

		work time	KB size	rest time	reps	
Round 3	JERK	45 sec.		60 sec.	L:	R:
	SNATCH	45 sec.		60 sec.	L:	R:
	BEHIND THE NECK SQUAT	30 sec.		60/30/15		
	WINDMILL (LEFT AND RIGHT)	30 sec.		60/30/15		
	DOUBLE KB LONG CYCLE CLEAN	30 sec.		60/30/15		
	STAGGERED PUSH-UP (EXPLOSIVE)	30 sec.		60/30/15		
	HIGH PLANK	30 sec.		60/30/15		

heart rate	comments:
start:	
end:	
5 min. post:	

Im Athletic 6 Month Workout Plan

DATE: _____

WARM UP: CHOOSE ONE WARM FROM THE DYNAMIC FLOW DRILL LIST

		work time	KB size	rest time	reps	
Round 1	LONG CYCLE BOTTOM UP JERK	45 sec.		60 sec.	L:	R:
	SNATCH	45 sec.		60 sec.	L:	R:
	DOUBLE SQUAT	30 sec.		60/30/15		
	BARBELL GET-UP SIT-UP	30 sec.		60/30/15		
	DOUBLE KB DEAD CLEAN	30 sec.		60/30/15		
	FIGURE 8 TO A HOLD	30 sec.		60/30/15		
	PUSH-UP	30 sec.		60/30/15		
	PLANK	30 sec.		60/30/15		

		work time	KB size	rest time	reps	
Round 2	PRESS	45 sec.		60 sec.	L:	R:
	SNATCH	45 sec.		60 sec.	L:	R:
	HAND 2 HAND SUMO DEADLIFT	30 sec.		60/30/15		
	SIDE BEND (LEFT AND RIGHT)	30 sec.		60/30/15		
	ALTERNATING CLEAN (DIP & SWITCH)	30 sec.		60/30/15		
	FIGURE 8 TO A HOLD	30 sec.		60/30/15		
	CLOSE GRIP PUSH-UP (MILITARY)	30 sec.		60/30/15		

		work time	KB size	rest time	reps	
Round 3	JERK	45 sec.		60 sec.	L:	R:
	SNATCH	45 sec.		60 sec.	L:	R:
	BEHIND THE NECK SQUAT	30 sec.		60/30/15		
	WINDMILL (LEFT AND RIGHT)	30 sec.		60/30/15		
	DOUBLE KB LONG CYCLE CLEAN	30 sec.		60/30/15		
	STAGGERED PUSH-UP (EXPLOSIVE)	30 sec.		60/30/15		
	HIGH PLANK	30 sec.		60/30/15		

heart rate	comments:
start:	
end:	
5 min. post:	

Im Athletic 6 Month Workout Plan

DATE: _____

WARM UP: CHOOSE ONE WARM FROM THE DYNAMIC FLOW DRILL LIST

		work time	KB size	rest time	reps	
Round 1	LONG CYCLE BOTTOM UP JERK	45 sec.		60 sec.	L:	R:
	SNATCH	45 sec.		60 sec.	L:	R:
	DOUBLE SQUAT	30 sec.		60/30/15		
	BARBELL GET-UP SIT-UP	30 sec.		60/30/15		
	DOUBLE KB DEAD CLEAN	30 sec.		60/30/15		
	FIGURE 8 TO A HOLD	30 sec.		60/30/15		
	PUSH-UP	30 sec.		60/30/15		
	PLANK	30 sec.		60/30/15		

		work time	KB size	rest time	reps	
Round 2	PRESS	45 sec.		60 sec.	L:	R:
	SNATCH	45 sec.		60 sec.	L:	R:
	HAND 2 HAND SUMO DEADLIFT	30 sec.		60/30/15		
	SIDE BEND (LEFT AND RIGHT)	30 sec.		60/30/15		
	ALTERNATING CLEAN (DIP & SWITCH)	30 sec.		60/30/15		
	FIGURE 8 TO A HOLD	30 sec.		60/30/15		
	CLOSE GRIP PUSH-UP (MILITARY)	30 sec.		60/30/15		

		work time	KB size	rest time	reps	
Round 3	JERK	45 sec.		60 sec.	L:	R:
	SNATCH	45 sec.		60 sec.	L:	R:
	BEHIND THE NECK SQUAT	30 sec.		60/30/15		
	WINDMILL (LEFT AND RIGHT)	30 sec.		60/30/15		
	DOUBLE KB LONG CYCLE CLEAN	30 sec.		60/30/15		
	STAGGERED PUSH-UP (EXPLOSIVE)	30 sec.		60/30/15		
	HIGH PLANK	30 sec.		60/30/15		

heart rate	comments:
start:	
end:	
5 min. post:	

Im Athletic 6 Month Workout Plan

DATE: _____

WARM UP: CHOOSE ONE WARM FROM THE DYNAMIC FLOW DRILL LIST

		work time	KB size	rest time	reps	
Round 1	LONG CYCLE BOTTOM UP JERK	45 sec.		60 sec.	L:	R:
	SNATCH	45 sec.		60 sec.	L:	R:
	DOUBLE SQUAT	30 sec.		60/30/15		
	BARBELL GET-UP SIT-UP	30 sec.		60/30/15		
	DOUBLE KB DEAD CLEAN	30 sec.		60/30/15		
	FIGURE 8 TO A HOLD	30 sec.		60/30/15		
	PUSH-UP	30 sec.		60/30/15		
	PLANK	30 sec.		60/30/15		

		work time	KB size	rest time	reps	
Round 2	PRESS	45 sec.		60 sec.	L:	R:
	SNATCH	45 sec.		60 sec.	L:	R:
	HAND 2 HAND SUMO DEADLIFT	30 sec.		60/30/15		
	SIDE BEND (LEFT AND RIGHT)	30 sec.		60/30/15		
	ALTERNATING CLEAN (DIP & SWITCH)	30 sec.		60/30/15		
	FIGURE 8 TO A HOLD	30 sec.		60/30/15		
	CLOSE GRIP PUSH-UP (MILITARY)	30 sec.		60/30/15		

		work time	KB size	rest time	reps	
Round 3	JERK	45 sec.		60 sec.	L:	R:
	SNATCH	45 sec.		60 sec.	L:	R:
	BEHIND THE NECK SQUAT	30 sec.		60/30/15		
	WINDMILL (LEFT AND RIGHT)	30 sec.		60/30/15		
	DOUBLE KB LONG CYCLE CLEAN	30 sec.		60/30/15		
	STAGGERED PUSH-UP (EXPLOSIVE)	30 sec.		60/30/15		
	HIGH PLANK	30 sec.		60/30/15		

heart rate	comments:
start:	
end:	
5 min. post:	

Im Athletic 6 Month Workout Plan

DATE: _____

WARM UP: CHOOSE ONE WARM FROM THE DYNAMIC FLOW DRILL LIST

		work time	KB size	rest time	reps	
Round 1	LONG CYCLE JERK	45 sec.		40 sec.	L:	R:
	1/2 SNATCH	45 sec.		40 sec.	L:	R:
	DOUBLE SQUAT	30 sec.		60/30/15		
	BARBELL GET-UP SIT-UP	30 sec.		60/30/15		
	DOUBLE KB DEAD CLEAN	30 sec.		60/30/15		
	FIGURE 8 TO A HOLD	30 sec.		60/30/15		
	PUSH-UP	30 sec.		60/30/15		
	PLANK	30 sec.		60/30/15		

		work time	KB size	rest time	reps	
Round 2	LONG CYCLE PRESS	45 sec.		40 sec.	L:	R:
	1/2 SNATCH	45 sec.		40 sec.	L:	R:
	HAND 2 HAND SUMO DEADLIFT	30 sec.		60/30/15		
	SIDE BEND (LEFT AND RIGHT)	30 sec.		60/30/15		
	ALTERNATING CLEAN (DIP & SWITCH)	30 sec.		60/30/15		
	FIGURE 8 TO A HOLD	30 sec.		60/30/15		
	CLOSE GRIP PUSH-UP (MILITARY)	30 sec.		60/30/15		

		work time	KB size	rest time	reps	
Round 3	JERK	45 sec.		40 sec.	L:	R:
	1/2 SNATCH	45 sec.		40 sec.	L:	R:
	BEHIND THE NECK SQUAT	30 sec.		60/30/15		
	WINDMILL (LEFT AND RIGHT)	30 sec.		60/30/15		
	DOUBLE KB LONG CYCLE CLEAN	30 sec.		60/30/15		
	STAGGERED PUSH-UP (EXPLOSIVE)	30 sec.		60/30/15		
	HIGH PLANK	30 sec.		60/30/15		

heart rate	comments:
start:	
end:	
5 min. post:	

Im Athletic 6 Month Workout Plan

DATE: _____

WARM UP: CHOOSE ONE WARM FROM THE DYNAMIC FLOW DRILL LIST

		work time	KB size	rest time	reps	
Round 1	LONG CYCLE JERK	45 sec.		40 sec.	L:	R:
	1/2 SNATCH	45 sec.		40 sec.	L:	R:
	DOUBLE SQUAT	30 sec.		60/30/15		
	BARBELL GET-UP SIT-UP	30 sec.		60/30/15		
	DOUBLE KB DEAD CLEAN	30 sec.		60/30/15		
	FIGURE 8 TO A HOLD	30 sec.		60/30/15		
	PUSH-UP	30 sec.		60/30/15		
	PLANK	30 sec.		60/30/15		

		work time	KB size	rest time	reps	
Round 2	LONG CYCLE PRESS	45 sec.		40 sec.	L:	R:
	1/2 SNATCH	45 sec.		40 sec.	L:	R:
	HAND 2 HAND SUMO DEADLIFT	30 sec.		60/30/15		
	SIDE BEND (LEFT AND RIGHT)	30 sec.		60/30/15		
	ALTERNATING CLEAN (DIP & SWITCH)	30 sec.		60/30/15		
	FIGURE 8 TO A HOLD	30 sec.		60/30/15		
	CLOSE GRIP PUSH-UP (MILITARY)	30 sec.		60/30/15		

		work time	KB size	rest time	reps	
Round 3	JERK	45 sec.		40 sec.	L:	R:
	1/2 SNATCH	45 sec.		40 sec.	L:	R:
	BEHIND THE NECK SQUAT	30 sec.		60/30/15		
	WINDMILL (LEFT AND RIGHT)	30 sec.		60/30/15		
	DOUBLE KB LONG CYCLE CLEAN	30 sec.		60/30/15		
	STAGGERED PUSH-UP (EXPLOSIVE)	30 sec.		60/30/15		
	HIGH PLANK	30 sec.		60/30/15		

heart rate	comments:
start:	
end:	
5 min. post:	

Im Athletic 6 Month Workout Plan

DATE: _____

WARM UP: CHOOSE ONE WARM FROM THE DYNAMIC FLOW DRILL LIST

Round 1		work time	KB size	rest time	reps	
	LONG CYCLE JERK	45 sec.		40 sec.	L:	R:
	1/2 SNATCH	45 sec.		40 sec.	L:	R:
	DOUBLE SQUAT	30 sec.		60/30/15		
	BARBELL GET-UP SIT-UP	30 sec.		60/30/15		
	DOUBLE KB DEAD CLEAN	30 sec.		60/30/15		
	FIGURE 8 TO A HOLD	30 sec.		60/30/15		
	PUSH-UP	30 sec.		60/30/15		
	PLANK	30 sec.		60/30/15		

Round 2		work time	KB size	rest time	reps	
	LONG CYCLE PRESS	45 sec.		40 sec.	L:	R:
	1/2 SNATCH	45 sec.		40 sec.	L:	R:
	HAND 2 HAND SUMO DEADLIFT	30 sec.		60/30/15		
	SIDE BEND (LEFT AND RIGHT)	30 sec.		60/30/15		
	ALTERNATING CLEAN (DIP & SWITCH)	30 sec.		60/30/15		
	FIGURE 8 TO A HOLD	30 sec.		60/30/15		
	CLOSE GRIP PUSH-UP (MILITARY)	30 sec.		60/30/15		

Round 3		work time	KB size	rest time	reps	
	JERK	45 sec.		40 sec.	L:	R:
	1/2 SNATCH	45 sec.		40 sec.	L:	R:
	BEHIND THE NECK SQUAT	30 sec.		60/30/15		
	WINDMILL (LEFT AND RIGHT)	30 sec.		60/30/15		
	DOUBLE KB LONG CYCLE CLEAN	30 sec.		60/30/15		
	STAGGERED PUSH-UP (EXPLOSIVE)	30 sec.		60/30/15		
	HIGH PLANK	30 sec.		60/30/15		

heart rate	comments:
start:	
end:	
5 min. post:	

Im Athletic 6 Month Workout Plan

DATE: _____

WARM UP: CHOOSE ONE WARM FROM THE DYNAMIC FLOW DRILL LIST

		work time	KB size	rest time	reps	
Round 1	LONG CYCLE JERK	45 sec.		40 sec.	L:	R:
	1/2 SNATCH	45 sec.		40 sec.	L:	R:
	DOUBLE SQUAT	30 sec.		60/30/15		
	BARBELL GET-UP SIT-UP	30 sec.		60/30/15		
	DOUBLE KB DEAD CLEAN	30 sec.		60/30/15		
	FIGURE 8 TO A HOLD	30 sec.		60/30/15		
	PUSH-UP	30 sec.		60/30/15		
	PLANK	30 sec.		60/30/15		

		work time	KB size	rest time	reps	
Round 2	LONG CYCLE PRESS	45 sec.		40 sec.	L:	R:
	1/2 SNATCH	45 sec.		40 sec.	L:	R:
	HAND 2 HAND SUMO DEADLIFT	30 sec.		60/30/15		
	SIDE BEND (LEFT AND RIGHT)	30 sec.		60/30/15		
	ALTERNATING CLEAN (DIP & SWITCH)	30 sec.		60/30/15		
	FIGURE 8 TO A HOLD	30 sec.		60/30/15		
	CLOSE GRIP PUSH-UP (MILITARY)	30 sec.		60/30/15		

		work time	KB size	rest time	reps	
Round 3	JERK	45 sec.		40 sec.	L:	R:
	1/2 SNATCH	45 sec.		40 sec.	L:	R:
	BEHIND THE NECK SQUAT	30 sec.		60/30/15		
	WINDMILL (LEFT AND RIGHT)	30 sec.		60/30/15		
	DOUBLE KB LONG CYCLE CLEAN	30 sec.		60/30/15		
	STAGGERED PUSH-UP (EXPLOSIVE)	30 sec.		60/30/15		
	HIGH PLANK	30 sec.		60/30/15		

heart rate	comments:
start:	
end:	
5 min. post:	

Im Athletic 6 Month Workout Plan

DATE: _____

MONTH: 2
WEEK: 4
DAY: 1

WARM UP: CHOOSE ONE WARM FROM THE DYNAMIC FLOW DRILL LIST

		work time	KB size	rest time	reps	
Round 1	PUSH PRESS	45 sec.		20 sec.	L:	R:
	SNATCH	45 sec.		20 sec.	L:	R:
	DOUBLE SQUAT	30 sec.		60/30/15		
	BARBELL GET-UP SIT-UP	30 sec.		60/30/15		
	DOUBLE KB DEAD CLEAN	30 sec.		60/30/15		
	FIGURE 8 TO A HOLD	30 sec.		60/30/15		
	PUSH-UP	30 sec.		60/30/15		
	PLANK	30 sec.		60/30/15		

		work time	KB size	rest time	reps	
Round 2	LONG CYCLE PRESS	45 sec.		20 sec.	L:	R:
	1/2 SNATCH	45 sec.		20 sec.	L:	R:
	HAND 2 HAND SUMO DEADLIFT	30 sec.		60/30/15		
	SIDE BEND (LEFT AND RIGHT)	30 sec.		60/30/15		
	ALTERNATING CLEAN (DIP & SWITCH)	30 sec.		60/30/15		
	FIGURE 8 TO A HOLD	30 sec.		60/30/15		
	CLOSE GRIP PUSH-UP (MILITARY)	30 sec.		60/30/15		

		work time	KB size	rest time	reps	
Round 3	LONG CYCLE BOTTOM UP PRESS	45 sec.		20 sec.	L:	R:
	1/2 SNATCH	45 sec.		20 sec.	L:	R:
	BEHIND THE NECK SQUAT	30 sec.		60/30/15		
	WINDMILL (LEFT AND RIGHT)	30 sec.		60/30/15		
	DOUBLE KB LONG CYCLE CLEAN	30 sec.		60/30/15		
	STAGGERED PUSH-UP (EXPLOSIVE)	30 sec.		60/30/15		
	HIGH PLANK	30 sec.		60/30/15		

heart rate	comments:
start:	
end:	
5 min. post:	

Im Athletic 6 Month Workout Plan

DATE: _____

WARM UP: CHOOSE ONE WARM FROM THE DYNAMIC FLOW DRILL LIST

		work time	KB size	rest time	reps	
Round 1	PUSH PRESS	45 sec.		20 sec.	L:	R:
	SNATCH	45 sec.		20 sec.	L:	R:
	DOUBLE SQUAT	30 sec.		60/30/15		
	BARBELL GET-UP SIT-UP	30 sec.		60/30/15		
	DOUBLE KB DEAD CLEAN	30 sec.		60/30/15		
	FIGURE 8 TO A HOLD	30 sec.		60/30/15		
	PUSH-UP	30 sec.		60/30/15		
	PLANK	30 sec.		60/30/15		

		work time	KB size	rest time	reps	
Round 2	LONG CYCLE PRESS	45 sec.		20 sec.	L:	R:
	1/2 SNATCH	45 sec.		20 sec.	L:	R:
	HAND 2 HAND SUMO DEADLIFT	30 sec.		60/30/15		
	SIDE BEND (LEFT AND RIGHT)	30 sec.		60/30/15		
	ALTERNATING CLEAN (DIP & SWITCH)	30 sec.		60/30/15		
	FIGURE 8 TO A HOLD	30 sec.		60/30/15		
	CLOSE GRIP PUSH-UP (MILITARY)	30 sec.		60/30/15		

		work time	KB size	rest time	reps	
Round 3	LONG CYCLE BOTTOM UP PRESS	45 sec.		20 sec.	L:	R:
	1/2 SNATCH	45 sec.		20 sec.	L:	R:
	BEHIND THE NECK SQUAT	30 sec.		60/30/15		
	WINDMILL (LEFT AND RIGHT)	30 sec.		60/30/15		
	DOUBLE KB LONG CYCLE CLEAN	30 sec.		60/30/15		
	STAGGERED PUSH-UP (EXPLOSIVE)	30 sec.		60/30/15		
	HIGH PLANK	30 sec.		60/30/15		

heart rate	comments:
start:	
end:	
5 min. post:	

Strength in Motion - Beyond ETK Workbook

DATE: _____

WARM UP: CHOOSE ONE WARM FROM THE DYNAMIC FLOW DRILL LIST

		work time	KB size	rest time	reps	
Round 1	PUSH PRESS	45 sec.		20 sec.	L:	R:
	SNATCH	45 sec.		20 sec.	L:	R:
	DOUBLE SQUAT	30 sec.		60/30/15		
	BARBELL GET-UP SIT-UP	30 sec.		60/30/15		
	DOUBLE KB DEAD CLEAN	30 sec.		60/30/15		
	FIGURE 8 TO A HOLD	30 sec.		60/30/15		
	PUSH-UP	30 sec.		60/30/15		
	PLANK	30 sec.		60/30/15		

		work time	KB size	rest time	reps	
Round 2	LONG CYCLE PRESS	45 sec.		20 sec.	L:	R:
	1/2 SNATCH	45 sec.		20 sec.	L:	R:
	HAND 2 HAND SUMO DEADLIFT	30 sec.		60/30/15		
	SIDE BEND (LEFT AND RIGHT)	30 sec.		60/30/15		
	ALTERNATING CLEAN (DIP & SWITCH)	30 sec.		60/30/15		
	FIGURE 8 TO A HOLD	30 sec.		60/30/15		
	CLOSE GRIP PUSH-UP (MILITARY)	30 sec.		60/30/15		

		work time	KB size	rest time	reps	
Round 3	LONG CYCLE BOTTOM UP PRESS	45 sec.		20 sec.	L:	R:
	1/2 SNATCH	45 sec.		20 sec.	L:	R:
	BEHIND THE NECK SQUAT	30 sec.		60/30/15		
	WINDMILL (LEFT AND RIGHT)	30 sec.		60/30/15		
	DOUBLE KB LONG CYCLE CLEAN	30 sec.		60/30/15		
	STAGGERED PUSH-UP (EXPLOSIVE)	30 sec.		60/30/15		
	HIGH PLANK	30 sec.		60/30/15		

heart rate	comments:
start:	
end:	
5 min. post:	

Im Athletic 6 Month Workout Plan

DATE: _____

WARM UP: CHOOSE ONE WARM FROM THE DYNAMIC FLOW DRILL LIST

		work time	KB size	rest time	reps	
Round 1	PUSH PRESS	45 sec.		20 sec.	L:	R:
	SNATCH	45 sec.		20 sec.	L:	R:
	DOUBLE SQUAT	30 sec.		60/30/15		
	BARBELL GET-UP SIT-UP	30 sec.		60/30/15		
	DOUBLE KB DEAD CLEAN	30 sec.		60/30/15		
	FIGURE 8 TO A HOLD	30 sec.		60/30/15		
	PUSH-UP	30 sec.		60/30/15		
	PLANK	30 sec.		60/30/15		

		work time	KB size	rest time	reps	
Round 2	LONG CYCLE PRESS	45 sec.		20 sec.	L:	R:
	1/2 SNATCH	45 sec.		20 sec.	L:	R:
	HAND 2 HAND SUMO DEADLIFT	30 sec.		60/30/15		
	SIDE BEND (LEFT AND RIGHT)	30 sec.		60/30/15		
	ALTERNATING CLEAN (DIP & SWITCH)	30 sec.		60/30/15		
	FIGURE 8 TO A HOLD	30 sec.		60/30/15		
	CLOSE GRIP PUSH-UP (MILITARY)	30 sec.		60/30/15		

		work time	KB size	rest time	reps	
Round 3	LONG CYCLE BOTTOM UP PRESS	45 sec.		20 sec.	L:	R:
	1/2 SNATCH	45 sec.		20 sec.	L:	R:
	BEHIND THE NECK SQUAT	30 sec.		60/30/15		
	WINDMILL (LEFT AND RIGHT)	30 sec.		60/30/15		
	DOUBLE KB LONG CYCLE CLEAN	30 sec.		60/30/15		
	STAGGERED PUSH-UP (EXPLOSIVE)	30 sec.		60/30/15		
	HIGH PLANK	30 sec.		60/30/15		

heart rate	comments:
start:	
end:	
5 min. post:	

You've finished month 2!

Benefit No. 1 to Kettlebell training:

Burns Fat in Less Time: Kettlebell training by its nature is metabolic, that is, it's based in cardio all while giving you the benefit of a strength training workout. Most of our workouts are performed "circuit style" with little to no break between rounds - offering maximum calorie burn in excess of 800-1000 calories for every 45-60 minute workout. That means no more stair stepper…

Im Athletic 6 Month Workout Plan

DATE: _____

WARM UP: CHOOSE ONE WARM FROM THE DYNAMIC FLOW DRILL LIST

Round 1		work time	KB size	rest time	reps	
	BOTTOM UP JERK	60 sec.		120 sec.	L:	R:
	1/2 SNATCH	60 sec.		120 sec.	L:	R:
	DOUBLE SQUAT	30 sec.		60/30/15		
	BARBELL GET-UP SIT-UP	30 sec.		60/30/15		
	DOUBLE KB DEAD CLEAN	30 sec.		60/30/15		
	FIGURE 8 TO A HOLD	30 sec.		60/30/15		
	PUSH-UP	30 sec.		60/30/15		
	PLANK	30 sec.		60/30/15		

Round 2		work time	KB size	rest time	reps	
	LONG CYCLE JERK	60 sec.		120 sec.	L:	R:
	1/2 SNATCH	60 sec.		120 sec.	L:	R:
	HAND 2 HAND SUMO DEADLIFT	30 sec.		60/30/15		
	SIDE BEND (LEFT AND RIGHT)	30 sec.		60/30/15		
	ALTERNATING CLEAN (DIP & SWITCH)	30 sec.		60/30/15		
	FIGURE 8 TO A HOLD	30 sec.		60/30/15		
	CLOSE GRIP PUSH-UP (MILITARY)	30 sec.		60/30/15		

Round 3		work time	KB size	rest time	reps	
	JERK	60 sec.		120 sec.	L:	R:
	SNATCH	60 sec.		120 sec.	L:	R:
	BEHIND THE NECK SQUAT	30 sec.		60/30/15		
	WINDMILL (LEFT AND RIGHT)	30 sec.		60/30/15		
	DOUBLE KB LONG CYCLE CLEAN	30 sec.		60/30/15		
	STAGGERED PUSH-UP (EXPLOSIVE)	30 sec.		60/30/15		
	HIGH PLANK	30 sec.		60/30/15		

heart rate	comments:
start:	
end:	
5 min. post:	

Im Athletic 6 Month Workout Plan

DATE: _____

MONTH: 3
WEEK: 1
DAY: 2

WARM UP: CHOOSE ONE WARM FROM THE DYNAMIC FLOW DRILL LIST

		work time	KB size	rest time	reps	
Round 1	BOTTOM UP JERK	60 sec.		120 sec.	L:	R:
	1/2 SNATCH	60 sec.		120 sec.	L:	R:
	DOUBLE SQUAT	30 sec.		60/30/15		
	BARBELL GET-UP SIT-UP	30 sec.		60/30/15		
	DOUBLE KB DEAD CLEAN	30 sec.		60/30/15		
	FIGURE 8 TO A HOLD	30 sec.		60/30/15		
	PUSH-UP	30 sec.		60/30/15		
	PLANK	30 sec.		60/30/15		

		work time	KB size	rest time	reps	
Round 2	LONG CYCLE JERK	60 sec.		120 sec.	L:	R:
	1/2 SNATCH	60 sec.		120 sec.	L:	R:
	HAND 2 HAND SUMO DEADLIFT	30 sec.		60/30/15		
	SIDE BEND (LEFT AND RIGHT)	30 sec.		60/30/15		
	ALTERNATING CLEAN (DIP & SWITCH)	30 sec.		60/30/15		
	FIGURE 8 TO A HOLD	30 sec.		60/30/15		
	CLOSE GRIP PUSH-UP (MILITARY)	30 sec.		60/30/15		

		work time	KB size	rest time	reps	
Round 3	JERK	60 sec.		120 sec.	L:	R:
	SNATCH	60 sec.		120 sec.	L:	R:
	BEHIND THE NECK SQUAT	30 sec.		60/30/15		
	WINDMILL (LEFT AND RIGHT)	30 sec.		60/30/15		
	DOUBLE KB LONG CYCLE CLEAN	30 sec.		60/30/15		
	STAGGERED PUSH-UP (EXPLOSIVE)	30 sec.		60/30/15		
	HIGH PLANK	30 sec.		60/30/15		

heart rate	comments:
start:	
end:	
5 min. post:	

Im Athletic 6 Month Workout Plan

DATE: _____

WARM UP: CHOOSE ONE WARM FROM THE DYNAMIC FLOW DRILL LIST

Round 1		work time	KB size	rest time	reps	
	BOTTOM UP JERK	60 sec.		120 sec.	L:	R:
	1/2 SNATCH	60 sec.		120 sec.	L:	R:
	DOUBLE SQUAT	30 sec.		60/30/15		
	BARBELL GET-UP SIT-UP	30 sec.		60/30/15		
	DOUBLE KB DEAD CLEAN	30 sec.		60/30/15		
	FIGURE 8 TO A HOLD	30 sec.		60/30/15		
	PUSH-UP	30 sec.		60/30/15		
	PLANK	30 sec.		60/30/15		

Round 2		work time	KB size	rest time	reps	
	LONG CYCLE JERK	60 sec.		120 sec.	L:	R:
	1/2 SNATCH	60 sec.		120 sec.	L:	R:
	HAND 2 HAND SUMO DEADLIFT	30 sec.		60/30/15		
	SIDE BEND (LEFT AND RIGHT)	30 sec.		60/30/15		
	ALTERNATING CLEAN (DIP & SWITCH)	30 sec.		60/30/15		
	FIGURE 8 TO A HOLD	30 sec.		60/30/15		
	CLOSE GRIP PUSH-UP (MILITARY)	30 sec.		60/30/15		

Round 3		work time	KB size	rest time	reps	
	JERK	60 sec.		120 sec.	L:	R:
	SNATCH	60 sec.		120 sec.	L:	R:
	BEHIND THE NECK SQUAT	30 sec.		60/30/15		
	WINDMILL (LEFT AND RIGHT)	30 sec.		60/30/15		
	DOUBLE KB LONG CYCLE CLEAN	30 sec.		60/30/15		
	STAGGERED PUSH-UP (EXPLOSIVE)	30 sec.		60/30/15		
	HIGH PLANK	30 sec.		60/30/15		

heart rate	comments:
start:	
end:	
5 min. post:	

Im Athletic 6 Month Workout Plan

DATE: _____

WARM UP: CHOOSE ONE WARM FROM THE DYNAMIC FLOW DRILL LIST

		work time	KB size	rest time	reps	
Round 1	BOTTOM UP JERK	60 sec.		120 sec.	L:	R:
	1/2 SNATCH	60 sec.		120 sec.	L:	R:
	DOUBLE SQUAT	30 sec.		60/30/15		
	BARBELL GET-UP SIT-UP	30 sec.		60/30/15		
	DOUBLE KB DEAD CLEAN	30 sec.		60/30/15		
	FIGURE 8 TO A HOLD	30 sec.		60/30/15		
	PUSH-UP	30 sec.		60/30/15		
	PLANK	30 sec.		60/30/15		

		work time	KB size	rest time	reps	
Round 2	LONG CYCLE JERK	60 sec.		120 sec.	L:	R:
	1/2 SNATCH	60 sec.		120 sec.	L:	R:
	HAND 2 HAND SUMO DEADLIFT	30 sec.		60/30/15		
	SIDE BEND (LEFT AND RIGHT)	30 sec.		60/30/15		
	ALTERNATING CLEAN (DIP & SWITCH)	30 sec.		60/30/15		
	FIGURE 8 TO A HOLD	30 sec.		60/30/15		
	CLOSE GRIP PUSH-UP (MILITARY)	30 sec.		60/30/15		

		work time	KB size	rest time	reps	
Round 3	JERK	60 sec.		120 sec.	L:	R:
	SNATCH	60 sec.		120 sec.	L:	R:
	BEHIND THE NECK SQUAT	30 sec.		60/30/15		
	WINDMILL (LEFT AND RIGHT)	30 sec.		60/30/15		
	DOUBLE KB LONG CYCLE CLEAN	30 sec.		60/30/15		
	STAGGERED PUSH-UP (EXPLOSIVE)	30 sec.		60/30/15		
	HIGH PLANK	30 sec.		60/30/15		

heart rate	comments:
start:	
end:	
5 min. post:	

Im Athletic 6 Month Workout Plan

DATE: _____

WARM UP: CHOOSE ONE WARM FROM THE DYNAMIC FLOW DRILL LIST

		work time	KB size	rest time	reps	
Round 1	BOTTOM UP PRESS	60 sec.		90 sec.	L:	R:
	SNATCH	60 sec.		90 sec.	L:	R:
	DOUBLE SQUAT	30 sec.		60/30/15		
	BARBELL GET-UP SIT-UP	30 sec.		60/30/15		
	DOUBLE KB DEAD CLEAN	30 sec.		60/30/15		
	FIGURE 8 TO A HOLD	30 sec.		60/30/15		
	PUSH-UP	30 sec.		60/30/15		
	PLANK	30 sec.		60/30/15		

		work time	KB size	rest time	reps	
Round 2	LONG CYCLE PRESS	60 sec.		90 sec.	L:	R:
	1/2 SNATCH	60 sec.		90 sec.	L:	R:
	HAND 2 HAND SUMO DEADLIFT	30 sec.		60/30/15		
	SIDE BEND (LEFT AND RIGHT)	30 sec.		60/30/15		
	ALTERNATING CLEAN (DIP & SWITCH)	30 sec.		60/30/15		
	FIGURE 8 TO A HOLD	30 sec.		60/30/15		
	CLOSE GRIP PUSH-UP (MILITARY)	30 sec.		60/30/15		

		work time	KB size	rest time	reps	
Round 3	LONG CYCLE JERK	60 sec.		90 sec.	L:	R:
	1/2 SNATCH	60 sec.		90 sec.	L:	R:
	BEHIND THE NECK SQUAT	30 sec.		60/30/15		
	WINDMILL (LEFT AND RIGHT)	30 sec.		60/30/15		
	DOUBLE KB LONG CYCLE CLEAN	30 sec.		60/30/15		
	STAGGERED PUSH-UP (EXPLOSIVE)	30 sec.		60/30/15		
	HIGH PLANK	30 sec.		60/30/15		

heart rate	comments:
start:	
end:	
5 min. post:	

Im Athletic 6 Month Workout Plan

DATE: _____

WARM UP: CHOOSE ONE WARM FROM THE DYNAMIC FLOW DRILL LIST

		work time	KB size	rest time	reps	
Round 1	BOTTOM UP PRESS	60 sec.		90 sec.	L:	R:
	SNATCH	60 sec.		90 sec.	L:	R:
	DOUBLE SQUAT	30 sec.		60/30/15		
	BARBELL GET-UP SIT-UP	30 sec.		60/30/15		
	DOUBLE KB DEAD CLEAN	30 sec.		60/30/15		
	FIGURE 8 TO A HOLD	30 sec.		60/30/15		
	PUSH-UP	30 sec.		60/30/15		
	PLANK	30 sec.		60/30/15		

		work time	KB size	rest time	reps	
Round 2	LONG CYCLE PRESS	60 sec.		90 sec.	L:	R:
	1/2 SNATCH	60 sec.		90 sec.	L:	R:
	HAND 2 HAND SUMO DEADLIFT	30 sec.		60/30/15		
	SIDE BEND (LEFT AND RIGHT)	30 sec.		60/30/15		
	ALTERNATING CLEAN (DIP & SWITCH)	30 sec.		60/30/15		
	FIGURE 8 TO A HOLD	30 sec.		60/30/15		
	CLOSE GRIP PUSH-UP (MILITARY)	30 sec.		60/30/15		

		work time	KB size	rest time	reps	
Round 3	LONG CYCLE JERK	60 sec.		90 sec.	L:	R:
	1/2 SNATCH	60 sec.		90 sec.	L:	R:
	BEHIND THE NECK SQUAT	30 sec.		60/30/15		
	WINDMILL (LEFT AND RIGHT)	30 sec.		60/30/15		
	DOUBLE KB LONG CYCLE CLEAN	30 sec.		60/30/15		
	STAGGERED PUSH-UP (EXPLOSIVE)	30 sec.		60/30/15		
	HIGH PLANK	30 sec.		60/30/15		

heart rate	comments:
start:	
end:	
5 min. post:	

Im Athletic 6 Month Workout Plan

DATE: _____

WARM UP: CHOOSE ONE WARM FROM THE DYNAMIC FLOW DRILL LIST

		work time	KB size	rest time	reps	
Round 1	BOTTOM UP PRESS	60 sec.		90 sec.	L:	R:
	SNATCH	60 sec.		90 sec.	L:	R:
	DOUBLE SQUAT	30 sec.		60/30/15		
	BARBELL GET-UP SIT-UP	30 sec.		60/30/15		
	DOUBLE KB DEAD CLEAN	30 sec.		60/30/15		
	FIGURE 8 TO A HOLD	30 sec.		60/30/15		
	PUSH-UP	30 sec.		60/30/15		
	PLANK	30 sec.		60/30/15		

		work time	KB size	rest time	reps	
Round 2	LONG CYCLE PRESS	60 sec.		90 sec.	L:	R:
	1/2 SNATCH	60 sec.		90 sec.	L:	R:
	HAND 2 HAND SUMO DEADLIFT	30 sec.		60/30/15		
	SIDE BEND (LEFT AND RIGHT)	30 sec.		60/30/15		
	ALTERNATING CLEAN (DIP & SWITCH)	30 sec.		60/30/15		
	FIGURE 8 TO A HOLD	30 sec.		60/30/15		
	CLOSE GRIP PUSH-UP (MILITARY)	30 sec.		60/30/15		

		work time	KB size	rest time	reps	
Round 3	LONG CYCLE JERK	60 sec.		90 sec.	L:	R:
	1/2 SNATCH	60 sec.		90 sec.	L:	R:
	BEHIND THE NECK SQUAT	30 sec.		60/30/15		
	WINDMILL (LEFT AND RIGHT)	30 sec.		60/30/15		
	DOUBLE KB LONG CYCLE CLEAN	30 sec.		60/30/15		
	STAGGERED PUSH-UP (EXPLOSIVE)	30 sec.		60/30/15		
	HIGH PLANK	30 sec.		60/30/15		

heart rate	comments:
start:	
end:	
5 min. post:	

Im Athletic 6 Month Workout Plan

DATE: _____

WARM UP: CHOOSE ONE WARM FROM THE DYNAMIC FLOW DRILL LIST

Round 1		work time	KB size	rest time	reps	
	BOTTOM UP PRESS	60 sec.		90 sec.	L:	R:
	SNATCH	60 sec.		90 sec.	L:	R:
	DOUBLE SQUAT	30 sec.		60/30/15		
	BARBELL GET-UP SIT-UP	30 sec.		60/30/15		
	DOUBLE KB DEAD CLEAN	30 sec.		60/30/15		
	FIGURE 8 TO A HOLD	30 sec.		60/30/15		
	PUSH-UP	30 sec.		60/30/15		
	PLANK	30 sec.		60/30/15		

Round 2		work time	KB size	rest time	reps	
	LONG CYCLE PRESS	60 sec.		90 sec.	L:	R:
	1/2 SNATCH	60 sec.		90 sec.	L:	R:
	HAND 2 HAND SUMO DEADLIFT	30 sec.		60/30/15		
	SIDE BEND (LEFT AND RIGHT)	30 sec.		60/30/15		
	ALTERNATING CLEAN (DIP & SWITCH)	30 sec.		60/30/15		
	FIGURE 8 TO A HOLD	30 sec.		60/30/15		
	CLOSE GRIP PUSH-UP (MILITARY)	30 sec.		60/30/15		

Round 3		work time	KB size	rest time	reps	
	LONG CYCLE JERK	60 sec.		90 sec.	L:	R:
	1/2 SNATCH	60 sec.		90 sec.	L:	R:
	BEHIND THE NECK SQUAT	30 sec.		60/30/15		
	WINDMILL (LEFT AND RIGHT)	30 sec.		60/30/15		
	DOUBLE KB LONG CYCLE CLEAN	30 sec.		60/30/15		
	STAGGERED PUSH-UP (EXPLOSIVE)	30 sec.		60/30/15		
	HIGH PLANK	30 sec.		60/30/15		

heart rate	comments:
start:	
end:	
5 min. post:	

Im Athletic 6 Month Workout Plan

DATE: _____

WARM UP: CHOOSE ONE WARM FROM THE DYNAMIC FLOW DRILL LIST

		work time	KB size	rest time	reps	
Round 1	LONG CYCLE JERK	60 sec.		60 sec.	L:	R:
	1/2 SNATCH	60 sec.		60 sec.	L:	R:
	DOUBLE SQUAT	30 sec.		60/30/15		
	BARBELL GET-UP SIT-UP	30 sec.		60/30/15		
	DOUBLE KB DEAD CLEAN	30 sec.		60/30/15		
	FIGURE 8 TO A HOLD	30 sec.		60/30/15		
	PUSH-UP	30 sec.		60/30/15		
	PLANK	30 sec.		60/30/15		

		work time	KB size	rest time	reps	
Round 2	LONG CYCLE JERK	60 sec.		60 sec.	L:	R:
	1/2 SNATCH	60 sec.		60 sec.	L:	R:
	HAND 2 HAND SUMO DEADLIFT	30 sec.		60/30/15		
	SIDE BEND (LEFT AND RIGHT)	30 sec.		60/30/15		
	ALTERNATING CLEAN (DIP & SWITCH)	30 sec.		60/30/15		
	FIGURE 8 TO A HOLD	30 sec.		60/30/15		
	CLOSE GRIP PUSH-UP (MILITARY)	30 sec.		60/30/15		

		work time	KB size	rest time	reps	
Round 3	LONG CYCLE JERK	60 sec.		60 sec.	L:	R:
	1/2 SNATCH	60 sec.		60 sec.	L:	R:
	BEHIND THE NECK SQUAT	30 sec.		60/30/15		
	WINDMILL (LEFT AND RIGHT)	30 sec.		60/30/15		
	DOUBLE KB LONG CYCLE CLEAN	30 sec.		60/30/15		
	STAGGERED PUSH-UP (EXPLOSIVE)	30 sec.		60/30/15		
	HIGH PLANK	30 sec.		60/30/15		

heart rate	comments:
start:	
end:	
5 min. post:	

Im Athletic 6 Month Workout Plan

DATE: _____

WARM UP: CHOOSE ONE WARM FROM THE DYNAMIC FLOW DRILL LIST

		work time	KB size	rest time	reps	
Round 1	LONG CYCLE JERK	60 sec.		60 sec.	L:	R:
	1/2 SNATCH	60 sec.		60 sec.	L:	R:
	DOUBLE SQUAT	30 sec.		60/30/15		
	BARBELL GET-UP SIT-UP	30 sec.		60/30/15		
	DOUBLE KB DEAD CLEAN	30 sec.		60/30/15		
	FIGURE 8 TO A HOLD	30 sec.		60/30/15		
	PUSH-UP	30 sec.		60/30/15		
	PLANK	30 sec.		60/30/15		

		work time	KB size	rest time	reps	
Round 2	LONG CYCLE JERK	60 sec.		60 sec.	L:	R:
	1/2 SNATCH	60 sec.		60 sec.	L:	R:
	HAND 2 HAND SUMO DEADLIFT	30 sec.		60/30/15		
	SIDE BEND (LEFT AND RIGHT)	30 sec.		60/30/15		
	ALTERNATING CLEAN (DIP & SWITCH)	30 sec.		60/30/15		
	FIGURE 8 TO A HOLD	30 sec.		60/30/15		
	CLOSE GRIP PUSH-UP (MILITARY)	30 sec.		60/30/15		

		work time	KB size	rest time	reps	
Round 3	LONG CYCLE JERK	60 sec.		60 sec.	L:	R:
	1/2 SNATCH	60 sec.		60 sec.	L:	R:
	BEHIND THE NECK SQUAT	30 sec.		60/30/15		
	WINDMILL (LEFT AND RIGHT)	30 sec.		60/30/15		
	DOUBLE KB LONG CYCLE CLEAN	30 sec.		60/30/15		
	STAGGERED PUSH-UP (EXPLOSIVE)	30 sec.		60/30/15		
	HIGH PLANK	30 sec.		60/30/15		

heart rate	comments:
start:	
end:	
5 min. post:	

Im Athletic 6 Month Workout Plan

DATE: _____

MONTH: 3
WEEK: 3
DAY: 3

WARM UP: CHOOSE ONE WARM FROM THE DYNAMIC FLOW DRILL LIST

		work time	KB size	rest time	reps	
Round 1	LONG CYCLE JERK	60 sec.		60 sec.	L:	R:
	1/2 SNATCH	60 sec.		60 sec.	L:	R:
	DOUBLE SQUAT	30 sec.		60/30/15		
	BARBELL GET-UP SIT-UP	30 sec.		60/30/15		
	DOUBLE KB DEAD CLEAN	30 sec.		60/30/15		
	FIGURE 8 TO A HOLD	30 sec.		60/30/15		
	PUSH-UP	30 sec.		60/30/15		
	PLANK	30 sec.		60/30/15		

		work time	KB size	rest time	reps	
Round 2	LONG CYCLE JERK	60 sec.		60 sec.	L:	R:
	1/2 SNATCH	60 sec.		60 sec.	L:	R:
	HAND 2 HAND SUMO DEADLIFT	30 sec.		60/30/15		
	SIDE BEND (LEFT AND RIGHT)	30 sec.		60/30/15		
	ALTERNATING CLEAN (DIP & SWITCH)	30 sec.		60/30/15		
	FIGURE 8 TO A HOLD	30 sec.		60/30/15		
	CLOSE GRIP PUSH-UP (MILITARY)	30 sec.		60/30/15		

		work time	KB size	rest time	reps	
Round 3	LONG CYCLE JERK	60 sec.		60 sec.	L:	R:
	1/2 SNATCH	60 sec.		60 sec.	L:	R:
	BEHIND THE NECK SQUAT	30 sec.		60/30/15		
	WINDMILL (LEFT AND RIGHT)	30 sec.		60/30/15		
	DOUBLE KB LONG CYCLE CLEAN	30 sec.		60/30/15		
	STAGGERED PUSH-UP (EXPLOSIVE)	30 sec.		60/30/15		
	HIGH PLANK	30 sec.		60/30/15		

heart rate	comments:
start:	
end:	
5 min. post:	

Im Athletic 6 Month Workout Plan

DATE: _____

WARM UP: CHOOSE ONE WARM FROM THE DYNAMIC FLOW DRILL LIST

		work time	KB size	rest time	reps	
Round 1	LONG CYCLE JERK	60 sec.		60 sec.	L:	R:
	1/2 SNATCH	60 sec.		60 sec.	L:	R:
	DOUBLE SQUAT	30 sec.		60/30/15		
	BARBELL GET-UP SIT-UP	30 sec.		60/30/15		
	DOUBLE KB DEAD CLEAN	30 sec.		60/30/15		
	FIGURE 8 TO A HOLD	30 sec.		60/30/15		
	PUSH-UP	30 sec.		60/30/15		
	PLANK	30 sec.		60/30/15		

		work time	KB size	rest time	reps	
Round 2	LONG CYCLE JERK	60 sec.		60 sec.	L:	R:
	1/2 SNATCH	60 sec.		60 sec.	L:	R:
	HAND 2 HAND SUMO DEADLIFT	30 sec.		60/30/15		
	SIDE BEND (LEFT AND RIGHT)	30 sec.		60/30/15		
	ALTERNATING CLEAN (DIP & SWITCH)	30 sec.		60/30/15		
	FIGURE 8 TO A HOLD	30 sec.		60/30/15		
	CLOSE GRIP PUSH-UP (MILITARY)	30 sec.		60/30/15		

		work time	KB size	rest time	reps	
Round 3	LONG CYCLE JERK	60 sec.		60 sec.	L:	R:
	1/2 SNATCH	60 sec.		60 sec.	L:	R:
	BEHIND THE NECK SQUAT	30 sec.		60/30/15		
	WINDMILL (LEFT AND RIGHT)	30 sec.		60/30/15		
	DOUBLE KB LONG CYCLE CLEAN	30 sec.		60/30/15		
	STAGGERED PUSH-UP (EXPLOSIVE)	30 sec.		60/30/15		
	HIGH PLANK	30 sec.		60/30/15		

heart rate	comments:
start:	
end:	
5 min. post:	

Im Athletic 6 Month Workout Plan

DATE: _____

WARM UP: CHOOSE ONE WARM FROM THE DYNAMIC FLOW DRILL LIST

		work time	KB size	rest time	reps	
Round 1	JERK	60 sec.		30 sec.	L:	R:
	SNATCH	60 sec.		30 sec.	L:	R:
	DOUBLE SQUAT	30 sec.		60/30/15		
	BARBELL GET-UP SIT-UP	30 sec.		60/30/15		
	DOUBLE KB DEAD CLEAN	30 sec.		60/30/15		
	FIGURE 8 TO A HOLD	30 sec.		60/30/15		
	PUSH-UP	30 sec.		60/30/15		
	PLANK	30 sec.		60/30/15		

		work time	KB size	rest time	reps	
Round 2	JERK	60 sec.		30 sec.	L:	R:
	SNATCH	60 sec.		30 sec.	L:	R:
	HAND 2 HAND SUMO DEADLIFT	30 sec.		60/30/15		
	SIDE BEND (LEFT AND RIGHT)	30 sec.		60/30/15		
	ALTERNATING CLEAN (DIP & SWITCH)	30 sec.		60/30/15		
	FIGURE 8 TO A HOLD	30 sec.		60/30/15		
	CLOSE GRIP PUSH-UP (MILITARY)	30 sec.		60/30/15		

		work time	KB size	rest time	reps	
Round 3	JERK	60 sec.		30 sec.	L:	R:
	SNATCH	60 sec.		30 sec.	L:	R:
	BEHIND THE NECK SQUAT	30 sec.		60/30/15		
	WINDMILL (LEFT AND RIGHT)	30 sec.		60/30/15		
	DOUBLE KB LONG CYCLE CLEAN	30 sec.		60/30/15		
	STAGGERED PUSH-UP (EXPLOSIVE)	30 sec.		60/30/15		
	HIGH PLANK	30 sec.		60/30/15		

heart rate	comments:
start:	
end:	
5 min. post:	

Im Athletic 6 Month Workout Plan

DATE: _____

WARM UP: CHOOSE ONE WARM FROM THE DYNAMIC FLOW DRILL LIST

		work time	KB size	rest time	reps	
Round 1	JERK	60 sec.		30 sec.	L:	R:
	SNATCH	60 sec.		30 sec.	L:	R:
	DOUBLE SQUAT	30 sec.		60/30/15		
	BARBELL GET-UP SIT-UP	30 sec.		60/30/15		
	DOUBLE KB DEAD CLEAN	30 sec.		60/30/15		
	FIGURE 8 TO A HOLD	30 sec.		60/30/15		
	PUSH-UP	30 sec.		60/30/15		
	PLANK	30 sec.		60/30/15		

		work time	KB size	rest time	reps	
Round 2	JERK	60 sec.		30 sec.	L:	R:
	SNATCH	60 sec.		30 sec.	L:	R:
	HAND 2 HAND SUMO DEADLIFT	30 sec.		60/30/15		
	SIDE BEND (LEFT AND RIGHT)	30 sec.		60/30/15		
	ALTERNATING CLEAN (DIP & SWITCH)	30 sec.		60/30/15		
	FIGURE 8 TO A HOLD	30 sec.		60/30/15		
	CLOSE GRIP PUSH-UP (MILITARY)	30 sec.		60/30/15		

		work time	KB size	rest time	reps	
Round 3	JERK	60 sec.		30 sec.	L:	R:
	SNATCH	60 sec.		30 sec.	L:	R:
	BEHIND THE NECK SQUAT	30 sec.		60/30/15		
	WINDMILL (LEFT AND RIGHT)	30 sec.		60/30/15		
	DOUBLE KB LONG CYCLE CLEAN	30 sec.		60/30/15		
	STAGGERED PUSH-UP (EXPLOSIVE)	30 sec.		60/30/15		
	HIGH PLANK	30 sec.		60/30/15		

heart rate	comments:
start:	
end:	
5 min. post:	

Im Athletic 6 Month Workout Plan

DATE: _____

MONTH: 3
WEEK: 4
DAY: 3

WARM UP: CHOOSE ONE WARM FROM THE DYNAMIC FLOW DRILL LIST

		work time	KB size	rest time	reps	
Round 1	JERK	60 sec.		30 sec.	L:	R:
	SNATCH	60 sec.		30 sec.	L:	R:
	DOUBLE SQUAT	30 sec.		60/30/15		
	BARBELL GET-UP SIT-UP	30 sec.		60/30/15		
	DOUBLE KB DEAD CLEAN	30 sec.		60/30/15		
	FIGURE 8 TO A HOLD	30 sec.		60/30/15		
	PUSH-UP	30 sec.		60/30/15		
	PLANK	30 sec.		60/30/15		

		work time	KB size	rest time	reps	
Round 2	JERK	60 sec.		30 sec.	L:	R:
	SNATCH	60 sec.		30 sec.	L:	R:
	HAND 2 HAND SUMO DEADLIFT	30 sec.		60/30/15		
	SIDE BEND (LEFT AND RIGHT)	30 sec.		60/30/15		
	ALTERNATING CLEAN (DIP & SWITCH)	30 sec.		60/30/15		
	FIGURE 8 TO A HOLD	30 sec.		60/30/15		
	CLOSE GRIP PUSH-UP (MILITARY)	30 sec.		60/30/15		

		work time	KB size	rest time	reps	
Round 3	JERK	60 sec.		30 sec.	L:	R:
	SNATCH	60 sec.		30 sec.	L:	R:
	BEHIND THE NECK SQUAT	30 sec.		60/30/15		
	WINDMILL (LEFT AND RIGHT)	30 sec.		60/30/15		
	DOUBLE KB LONG CYCLE CLEAN	30 sec.		60/30/15		
	STAGGERED PUSH-UP (EXPLOSIVE)	30 sec.		60/30/15		
	HIGH PLANK	30 sec.		60/30/15		

heart rate	comments:
start:	
end:	
5 min. post:	

Im Athletic 6 Month Workout Plan

DATE: _____

WARM UP: CHOOSE ONE WARM FROM THE DYNAMIC FLOW DRILL LIST

		work time	KB size	rest time	reps	
Round 1	JERK	60 sec.		30 sec.	L:	R:
	SNATCH	60 sec.		30 sec.	L:	R:
	DOUBLE SQUAT	30 sec.		60/30/15		
	BARBELL GET-UP SIT-UP	30 sec.		60/30/15		
	DOUBLE KB DEAD CLEAN	30 sec.		60/30/15		
	FIGURE 8 TO A HOLD	30 sec.		60/30/15		
	PUSH-UP	30 sec.		60/30/15		
	PLANK	30 sec.		60/30/15		

		work time	KB size	rest time	reps	
Round 2	JERK	60 sec.		30 sec.	L:	R:
	SNATCH	60 sec.		30 sec.	L:	R:
	HAND 2 HAND SUMO DEADLIFT	30 sec.		60/30/15		
	SIDE BEND (LEFT AND RIGHT)	30 sec.		60/30/15		
	ALTERNATING CLEAN (DIP & SWITCH)	30 sec.		60/30/15		
	FIGURE 8 TO A HOLD	30 sec.		60/30/15		
	CLOSE GRIP PUSH-UP (MILITARY)	30 sec.		60/30/15		

		work time	KB size	rest time	reps	
Round 3	JERK	60 sec.		30 sec.	L:	R:
	SNATCH	60 sec.		30 sec.	L:	R:
	BEHIND THE NECK SQUAT	30 sec.		60/30/15		
	WINDMILL (LEFT AND RIGHT)	30 sec.		60/30/15		
	DOUBLE KB LONG CYCLE CLEAN	30 sec.		60/30/15		
	STAGGERED PUSH-UP (EXPLOSIVE)	30 sec.		60/30/15		
	HIGH PLANK	30 sec.		60/30/15		

heart rate	comments:
start:	
end:	
5 min. post:	

Im Athletic 6 Month Workout Plan

DATE: _____

WARM UP: CHOOSE ONE WARM FROM THE DYNAMIC FLOW DRILL LIST

		work time	KB size	rest time	reps	
Round 1	JERK	90 sec.		180 sec.	L:	R:
	1/2 SNATCH	90 sec.		180 sec.	L:	R:
	DOUBLE SQUAT	30 sec.		60/30/15		
	BARBELL GET-UP SIT-UP	30 sec.		60/30/15		
	DOUBLE KB DEAD CLEAN	30 sec.		60/30/15		
	FIGURE 8 TO A HOLD	30 sec.		60/30/15		
	PUSH-UP	30 sec.		60/30/15		
	PLANK	30 sec.		60/30/15		

		work time	KB size	rest time	reps	
Round 2	PRESS	90 sec.		180 sec.	L:	R:
	1/2 SNATCH	90 sec.		180 sec.	L:	R:
	HAND 2 HAND SUMO DEADLIFT	30 sec.		60/30/15		
	SIDE BEND (LEFT AND RIGHT)	30 sec.		60/30/15		
	ALTERNATING CLEAN (DIP & SWITCH)	30 sec.		60/30/15		
	FIGURE 8 TO A HOLD	30 sec.		60/30/15		
	CLOSE GRIP PUSH-UP (MILITARY)	30 sec.		60/30/15		

		work time	KB size	rest time	reps	
Round 3	JERK	90 sec.		180 sec.	L:	R:
	SNATCH	90 sec.		180 sec.	L:	R:
	BEHIND THE NECK SQUAT	30 sec.		60/30/15		
	WINDMILL (LEFT AND RIGHT)	30 sec.		60/30/15		
	DOUBLE KB LONG CYCLE CLEAN	30 sec.		60/30/15		
	STAGGERED PUSH-UP (EXPLOSIVE)	30 sec.		60/30/15		
	HIGH PLANK	30 sec.		60/30/15		

heart rate	comments:
start:	
end:	
5 min. post:	

Im Athletic 6 Month Workout Plan

DATE: _____

WARM UP: CHOOSE ONE WARM FROM THE DYNAMIC FLOW DRILL LIST

		work time	KB size	rest time	reps	
Round 1	JERK	90 sec.		180 sec.	L:	R:
	1/2 SNATCH	90 sec.		180 sec.	L:	R:
	DOUBLE SQUAT	30 sec.		60/30/15		
	BARBELL GET-UP SIT-UP	30 sec.		60/30/15		
	DOUBLE KB DEAD CLEAN	30 sec.		60/30/15		
	FIGURE 8 TO A HOLD	30 sec.		60/30/15		
	PUSH-UP	30 sec.		60/30/15		
	PLANK	30 sec.		60/30/15		

		work time	KB size	rest time	reps	
Round 2	PRESS	90 sec.		180 sec.	L:	R:
	1/2 SNATCH	90 sec.		180 sec.	L:	R:
	HAND 2 HAND SUMO DEADLIFT	30 sec.		60/30/15		
	SIDE BEND (LEFT AND RIGHT)	30 sec.		60/30/15		
	ALTERNATING CLEAN (DIP & SWITCH)	30 sec.		60/30/15		
	FIGURE 8 TO A HOLD	30 sec.		60/30/15		
	CLOSE GRIP PUSH-UP (MILITARY)	30 sec.		60/30/15		

		work time	KB size	rest time	reps	
Round 3	JERK	90 sec.		180 sec.	L:	R:
	SNATCH	90 sec.		180 sec.	L:	R:
	BEHIND THE NECK SQUAT	30 sec.		60/30/15		
	WINDMILL (LEFT AND RIGHT)	30 sec.		60/30/15		
	DOUBLE KB LONG CYCLE CLEAN	30 sec.		60/30/15		
	STAGGERED PUSH-UP (EXPLOSIVE)	30 sec.		60/30/15		
	HIGH PLANK	30 sec.		60/30/15		

heart rate	comments:
start:	
end:	
5 min. post:	

Im Athletic 6 Month Workout Plan

DATE: _____

MONTH: 4
WEEK: 1
DAY: 3

WARM UP: CHOOSE ONE WARM FROM THE DYNAMIC FLOW DRILL LIST

		work time	KB size	rest time	reps	
Round 1	JERK	90 sec.		180 sec.	L:	R:
	1/2 SNATCH	90 sec.		180 sec.	L:	R:
	DOUBLE SQUAT	30 sec.		60/30/15		
	BARBELL GET-UP SIT-UP	30 sec.		60/30/15		
	DOUBLE KB DEAD CLEAN	30 sec.		60/30/15		
	FIGURE 8 TO A HOLD	30 sec.		60/30/15		
	PUSH-UP	30 sec.		60/30/15		
	PLANK	30 sec.		60/30/15		

		work time	KB size	rest time	reps	
Round 2	PRESS	90 sec.		180 sec.	L:	R:
	1/2 SNATCH	90 sec.		180 sec.	L:	R:
	HAND 2 HAND SUMO DEADLIFT	30 sec.		60/30/15		
	SIDE BEND (LEFT AND RIGHT)	30 sec.		60/30/15		
	ALTERNATING CLEAN (DIP & SWITCH)	30 sec.		60/30/15		
	FIGURE 8 TO A HOLD	30 sec.		60/30/15		
	CLOSE GRIP PUSH-UP (MILITARY)	30 sec.		60/30/15		

		work time	KB size	rest time	reps	
Round 3	JERK	90 sec.		180 sec.	L:	R:
	SNATCH	90 sec.		180 sec.	L:	R:
	BEHIND THE NECK SQUAT	30 sec.		60/30/15		
	WINDMILL (LEFT AND RIGHT)	30 sec.		60/30/15		
	DOUBLE KB LONG CYCLE CLEAN	30 sec.		60/30/15		
	STAGGERED PUSH-UP (EXPLOSIVE)	30 sec.		60/30/15		
	HIGH PLANK	30 sec.		60/30/15		

heart rate	comments:
start:	
end:	
5 min. post:	

Im Athletic 6 Month Workout Plan

DATE: _____

WARM UP: CHOOSE ONE WARM FROM THE DYNAMIC FLOW DRILL LIST

		work time	KB size	rest time	reps	
Round 1	JERK	90 sec.		180 sec.	L:	R:
	1/2 SNATCH	90 sec.		180 sec.	L:	R:
	DOUBLE SQUAT	30 sec.		60/30/15		
	BARBELL GET-UP SIT-UP	30 sec.		60/30/15		
	DOUBLE KB DEAD CLEAN	30 sec.		60/30/15		
	FIGURE 8 TO A HOLD	30 sec.		60/30/15		
	PUSH-UP	30 sec.		60/30/15		
	PLANK	30 sec.		60/30/15		

		work time	KB size	rest time	reps	
Round 2	PRESS	90 sec.		180 sec.	L:	R:
	1/2 SNATCH	90 sec.		180 sec.	L:	R:
	HAND 2 HAND SUMO DEADLIFT	30 sec.		60/30/15		
	SIDE BEND (LEFT AND RIGHT)	30 sec.		60/30/15		
	ALTERNATING CLEAN (DIP & SWITCH)	30 sec.		60/30/15		
	FIGURE 8 TO A HOLD	30 sec.		60/30/15		
	CLOSE GRIP PUSH-UP (MILITARY)	30 sec.		60/30/15		

		work time	KB size	rest time	reps	
Round 3	JERK	90 sec.		180 sec.	L:	R:
	SNATCH	90 sec.		180 sec.	L:	R:
	BEHIND THE NECK SQUAT	30 sec.		60/30/15		
	WINDMILL (LEFT AND RIGHT)	30 sec.		60/30/15		
	DOUBLE KB LONG CYCLE CLEAN	30 sec.		60/30/15		
	STAGGERED PUSH-UP (EXPLOSIVE)	30 sec.		60/30/15		
	HIGH PLANK	30 sec.		60/30/15		

heart rate	comments:
start:	
end:	
5 min. post:	

Im Athletic 6 Month Workout Plan

DATE: _____

WARM UP: CHOOSE ONE WARM FROM THE DYNAMIC FLOW DRILL LIST

		work time	KB size	rest time	reps	
Round 1	BOTTOM UP PUSH PRESS	90 sec.		120 sec.	L:	R:
	1/2 SNATCH	90 sec.		120 sec.	L:	R:
	DOUBLE SQUAT	30 sec.		60/30/15		
	BARBELL GET-UP SIT-UP	30 sec.		60/30/15		
	DOUBLE KB DEAD CLEAN	30 sec.		60/30/15		
	FIGURE 8 TO A HOLD	30 sec.		60/30/15		
	PUSH-UP	30 sec.		60/30/15		
	PLANK	30 sec.		60/30/15		

		work time	KB size	rest time	reps	
Round 2	LONG CYCLE JERK	90 sec.		120 sec.	L:	R:
	SNATCH	90 sec.		120 sec.	L:	R:
	HAND 2 HAND SUMO DEADLIFT	30 sec.		60/30/15		
	SIDE BEND (LEFT AND RIGHT)	30 sec.		60/30/15		
	ALTERNATING CLEAN (DIP & SWITCH)	30 sec.		60/30/15		
	FIGURE 8 TO A HOLD	30 sec.		60/30/15		
	CLOSE GRIP PUSH-UP (MILITARY)	30 sec.		60/30/15		

		work time	KB size	rest time	reps	
Round 3	JERK	90 sec.		120 sec.	L:	R:
	SNATCH	90 sec.		120 sec.	L:	R:
	BEHIND THE NECK SQUAT	30 sec.		60/30/15		
	WINDMILL (LEFT AND RIGHT)	30 sec.		60/30/15		
	DOUBLE KB LONG CYCLE CLEAN	30 sec.		60/30/15		
	STAGGERED PUSH-UP (EXPLOSIVE)	30 sec.		60/30/15		
	HIGH PLANK	30 sec.		60/30/15		

heart rate	comments:
start:	
end:	
5 min. post:	

Im Athletic 6 Month Workout Plan

DATE: _____

WARM UP: CHOOSE ONE WARM FROM THE DYNAMIC FLOW DRILL LIST

Round 1		work time	KB size	rest time	reps	
	BOTTOM UP PUSH PRESS	90 sec.		120 sec.	L:	R:
	1/2 SNATCH	90 sec.		120 sec.	L:	R:
	DOUBLE SQUAT	30 sec.		60/30/15		
	BARBELL GET-UP SIT-UP	30 sec.		60/30/15		
	DOUBLE KB DEAD CLEAN	30 sec.		60/30/15		
	FIGURE 8 TO A HOLD	30 sec.		60/30/15		
	PUSH-UP	30 sec.		60/30/15		
	PLANK	30 sec.		60/30/15		

Round 2		work time	KB size	rest time	reps	
	LONG CYCLE JERK	90 sec.		120 sec.	L:	R:
	SNATCH	90 sec.		120 sec.	L:	R:
	HAND 2 HAND SUMO DEADLIFT	30 sec.		60/30/15		
	SIDE BEND (LEFT AND RIGHT)	30 sec.		60/30/15		
	ALTERNATING CLEAN (DIP & SWITCH)	30 sec.		60/30/15		
	FIGURE 8 TO A HOLD	30 sec.		60/30/15		
	CLOSE GRIP PUSH-UP (MILITARY)	30 sec.		60/30/15		

Round 3		work time	KB size	rest time	reps	
	JERK	90 sec.		120 sec.	L:	R:
	SNATCH	90 sec.		120 sec.	L:	R:
	BEHIND THE NECK SQUAT	30 sec.		60/30/15		
	WINDMILL (LEFT AND RIGHT)	30 sec.		60/30/15		
	DOUBLE KB LONG CYCLE CLEAN	30 sec.		60/30/15		
	STAGGERED PUSH-UP (EXPLOSIVE)	30 sec.		60/30/15		
	HIGH PLANK	30 sec.		60/30/15		

heart rate	comments:
start:	
end:	
5 min. post:	

Im Athletic 6 Month Workout Plan

DATE: _____

WARM UP: CHOOSE ONE WARM FROM THE DYNAMIC FLOW DRILL LIST

		work time	KB size	rest time	reps	
Round 1	BOTTOM UP PUSH PRESS	90 sec.		120 sec.	L:	R:
	1/2 SNATCH	90 sec.		120 sec.	L:	R:
	DOUBLE SQUAT	30 sec.		60/30/15		
	BARBELL GET-UP SIT-UP	30 sec.		60/30/15		
	DOUBLE KB DEAD CLEAN	30 sec.		60/30/15		
	FIGURE 8 TO A HOLD	30 sec.		60/30/15		
	PUSH-UP	30 sec.		60/30/15		
	PLANK	30 sec.		60/30/15		

		work time	KB size	rest time	reps	
Round 2	LONG CYCLE JERK	90 sec.		120 sec.	L:	R:
	SNATCH	90 sec.		120 sec.	L:	R:
	HAND 2 HAND SUMO DEADLIFT	30 sec.		60/30/15		
	SIDE BEND (LEFT AND RIGHT)	30 sec.		60/30/15		
	ALTERNATING CLEAN (DIP & SWITCH)	30 sec.		60/30/15		
	FIGURE 8 TO A HOLD	30 sec.		60/30/15		
	CLOSE GRIP PUSH-UP (MILITARY)	30 sec.		60/30/15		

		work time	KB size	rest time	reps	
Round 3	JERK	90 sec.		120 sec.	L:	R:
	SNATCH	90 sec.		120 sec.	L:	R:
	BEHIND THE NECK SQUAT	30 sec.		60/30/15		
	WINDMILL (LEFT AND RIGHT)	30 sec.		60/30/15		
	DOUBLE KB LONG CYCLE CLEAN	30 sec.		60/30/15		
	STAGGERED PUSH-UP (EXPLOSIVE)	30 sec.		60/30/15		
	HIGH PLANK	30 sec.		60/30/15		

heart rate	comments:
start:	
end:	
5 min. post:	

Im Athletic 6 Month Workout Plan

DATE: _____

MONTH: 4
WEEK: 2
DAY: 4

WARM UP: CHOOSE ONE WARM FROM THE DYNAMIC FLOW DRILL LIST

		work time	KB size	rest time	reps	
Round 1	BOTTOM UP PUSH PRESS	90 sec.		120 sec.	L:	R:
	1/2 SNATCH	90 sec.		120 sec.	L:	R:
	DOUBLE SQUAT	30 sec.		60/30/15		
	BARBELL GET-UP SIT-UP	30 sec.		60/30/15		
	DOUBLE KB DEAD CLEAN	30 sec.		60/30/15		
	FIGURE 8 TO A HOLD	30 sec.		60/30/15		
	PUSH-UP	30 sec.		60/30/15		
	PLANK	30 sec.		60/30/15		

		work time	KB size	rest time	reps	
Round 2	LONG CYCLE JERK	90 sec.		120 sec.	L:	R:
	SNATCH	90 sec.		120 sec.	L:	R:
	HAND 2 HAND SUMO DEADLIFT	30 sec.		60/30/15		
	SIDE BEND (LEFT AND RIGHT)	30 sec.		60/30/15		
	ALTERNATING CLEAN (DIP & SWITCH)	30 sec.		60/30/15		
	FIGURE 8 TO A HOLD	30 sec.		60/30/15		
	CLOSE GRIP PUSH-UP (MILITARY)	30 sec.		60/30/15		

		work time	KB size	rest time	reps	
Round 3	JERK	90 sec.		120 sec.	L:	R:
	SNATCH	90 sec.		120 sec.	L:	R:
	BEHIND THE NECK SQUAT	30 sec.		60/30/15		
	WINDMILL (LEFT AND RIGHT)	30 sec.		60/30/15		
	DOUBLE KB LONG CYCLE CLEAN	30 sec.		60/30/15		
	STAGGERED PUSH-UP (EXPLOSIVE)	30 sec.		60/30/15		
	HIGH PLANK	30 sec.		60/30/15		

heart rate	comments:
start:	
end:	
5 min. post:	

Im Athletic 6 Month Workout Plan

DATE: _____

WARM UP: CHOOSE ONE WARM FROM THE DYNAMIC FLOW DRILL LIST

		work time	KB size	rest time	reps	
Round 1	LONG CYCLE PUSH PRESS	90 sec.		90 sec.	L:	R:
	1/2 SNATCH	90 sec.		90 sec.	L:	R:
	DOUBLE SQUAT	30 sec.		60/30/15		
	BARBELL GET-UP SIT-UP	30 sec.		60/30/15		
	DOUBLE KB DEAD CLEAN	30 sec.		60/30/15		
	FIGURE 8 TO A HOLD	30 sec.		60/30/15		
	PUSH-UP	30 sec.		60/30/15		
	PLANK	30 sec.		60/30/15		

		work time	KB size	rest time	reps	
Round 2	BOTTOM UP JERK	90 sec.		90 sec.	L:	R:
	SNATCH	90 sec.		90 sec.	L:	R:
	HAND 2 HAND SUMO DEADLIFT	30 sec.		60/30/15		
	SIDE BEND (LEFT AND RIGHT)	30 sec.		60/30/15		
	ALTERNATING CLEAN (DIP & SWITCH)	30 sec.		60/30/15		
	FIGURE 8 TO A HOLD	30 sec.		60/30/15		
	CLOSE GRIP PUSH-UP (MILITARY)	30 sec.		60/30/15		

		work time	KB size	rest time	reps	
Round 3	JERK	90 sec.		90 sec.	L:	R:
	SNATCH	90 sec.		90 sec.	L:	R:
	BEHIND THE NECK SQUAT	30 sec.		60/30/15		
	WINDMILL (LEFT AND RIGHT)	30 sec.		60/30/15		
	DOUBLE KB LONG CYCLE CLEAN	30 sec.		60/30/15		
	STAGGERED PUSH-UP (EXPLOSIVE)	30 sec.		60/30/15		
	HIGH PLANK	30 sec.		60/30/15		

heart rate	comments:
start:	
end:	
5 min. post:	

Im Athletic 6 Month Workout Plan

DATE: _____

MONTH: 4
WEEK: 3
DAY: 2

WARM UP: CHOOSE ONE WARM FROM THE DYNAMIC FLOW DRILL LIST

Round 1

		work time	KB size	rest time	reps	
	LONG CYCLE PUSH PRESS	90 sec.		90 sec.	L:	R:
	1/2 SNATCH	90 sec.		90 sec.	L:	R:
	DOUBLE SQUAT	30 sec.		60/30/15		
	BARBELL GET-UP SIT-UP	30 sec.		60/30/15		
	DOUBLE KB DEAD CLEAN	30 sec.		60/30/15		
	FIGURE 8 TO A HOLD	30 sec.		60/30/15		
	PUSH-UP	30 sec.		60/30/15		
	PLANK	30 sec.		60/30/15		

Round 2

		work time	KB size	rest time	reps	
	BOTTOM UP JERK	90 sec.		90 sec.	L:	R:
	SNATCH	90 sec.		90 sec.	L:	R:
	HAND 2 HAND SUMO DEADLIFT	30 sec.		60/30/15		
	SIDE BEND (LEFT AND RIGHT)	30 sec.		60/30/15		
	ALTERNATING CLEAN (DIP & SWITCH)	30 sec.		60/30/15		
	FIGURE 8 TO A HOLD	30 sec.		60/30/15		
	CLOSE GRIP PUSH-UP (MILITARY)	30 sec.		60/30/15		

Round 3

		work time	KB size	rest time	reps	
	JERK	90 sec.		90 sec.	L:	R:
	SNATCH	90 sec.		90 sec.	L:	R:
	BEHIND THE NECK SQUAT	30 sec.		60/30/15		
	WINDMILL (LEFT AND RIGHT)	30 sec.		60/30/15		
	DOUBLE KB LONG CYCLE CLEAN	30 sec.		60/30/15		
	STAGGERED PUSH-UP (EXPLOSIVE)	30 sec.		60/30/15		
	HIGH PLANK	30 sec.		60/30/15		

heart rate	comments:
start:	
end:	
5 min. post:	

Im Athletic 6 Month Workout Plan

DATE: _____

WARM UP: CHOOSE ONE WARM FROM THE DYNAMIC FLOW DRILL LIST

		work time	KB size	rest time	reps	
Round 1	LONG CYCLE PUSH PRESS	90 sec.		90 sec.	L:	R:
	1/2 SNATCH	90 sec.		90 sec.	L:	R:
	DOUBLE SQUAT	30 sec.		60/30/15		
	BARBELL GET-UP SIT-UP	30 sec.		60/30/15		
	DOUBLE KB DEAD CLEAN	30 sec.		60/30/15		
	FIGURE 8 TO A HOLD	30 sec.		60/30/15		
	PUSH-UP	30 sec.		60/30/15		
	PLANK	30 sec.		60/30/15		

		work time	KB size	rest time	reps	
Round 2	BOTTOM UP JERK	90 sec.		90 sec.	L:	R:
	SNATCH	90 sec.		90 sec.	L:	R:
	HAND 2 HAND SUMO DEADLIFT	30 sec.		60/30/15		
	SIDE BEND (LEFT AND RIGHT)	30 sec.		60/30/15		
	ALTERNATING CLEAN (DIP & SWITCH)	30 sec.		60/30/15		
	FIGURE 8 TO A HOLD	30 sec.		60/30/15		
	CLOSE GRIP PUSH-UP (MILITARY)	30 sec.		60/30/15		

		work time	KB size	rest time	reps	
Round 3	JERK	90 sec.		90 sec.	L:	R:
	SNATCH	90 sec.		90 sec.	L:	R:
	BEHIND THE NECK SQUAT	30 sec.		60/30/15		
	WINDMILL (LEFT AND RIGHT)	30 sec.		60/30/15		
	DOUBLE KB LONG CYCLE CLEAN	30 sec.		60/30/15		
	STAGGERED PUSH-UP (EXPLOSIVE)	30 sec.		60/30/15		
	HIGH PLANK	30 sec.		60/30/15		

heart rate	comments:
start:	
end:	
5 min. post:	

Im Athletic 6 Month Workout Plan

DATE: _____

WARM UP: CHOOSE ONE WARM FROM THE DYNAMIC FLOW DRILL LIST

		work time	KB size	rest time	reps	
Round 1	LONG CYCLE PUSH PRESS	90 sec.		90 sec.	L:	R:
	1/2 SNATCH	90 sec.		90 sec.	L:	R:
	DOUBLE SQUAT	30 sec.		60/30/15		
	BARBELL GET-UP SIT-UP	30 sec.		60/30/15		
	DOUBLE KB DEAD CLEAN	30 sec.		60/30/15		
	FIGURE 8 TO A HOLD	30 sec.		60/30/15		
	PUSH-UP	30 sec.		60/30/15		
	PLANK	30 sec.		60/30/15		

		work time	KB size	rest time	reps	
Round 2	BOTTOM UP JERK	90 sec.		90 sec.	L:	R:
	SNATCH	90 sec.		90 sec.	L:	R:
	HAND 2 HAND SUMO DEADLIFT	30 sec.		60/30/15		
	SIDE BEND (LEFT AND RIGHT)	30 sec.		60/30/15		
	ALTERNATING CLEAN (DIP & SWITCH)	30 sec.		60/30/15		
	FIGURE 8 TO A HOLD	30 sec.		60/30/15		
	CLOSE GRIP PUSH-UP (MILITARY)	30 sec.		60/30/15		

		work time	KB size	rest time	reps	
Round 3	JERK	90 sec.		90 sec.	L:	R:
	SNATCH	90 sec.		90 sec.	L:	R:
	BEHIND THE NECK SQUAT	30 sec.		60/30/15		
	WINDMILL (LEFT AND RIGHT)	30 sec.		60/30/15		
	DOUBLE KB LONG CYCLE CLEAN	30 sec.		60/30/15		
	STAGGERED PUSH-UP (EXPLOSIVE)	30 sec.		60/30/15		
	HIGH PLANK	30 sec.		60/30/15		

heart rate	comments:
start:	
end:	
5 min. post:	

Im Athletic 6 Month Workout Plan

DATE: _____

WARM UP: CHOOSE ONE WARM FROM THE DYNAMIC FLOW DRILL LIST

		work time	KB size	rest time	reps	
Round 1	LONG CYCLE PRESS	90 sec.		45 sec.	L:	R:
	SNATCH	90 sec.		45 sec.	L:	R:
	DOUBLE SQUAT	30 sec.		60/30/15		
	BARBELL GET-UP SIT-UP	30 sec.		60/30/15		
	DOUBLE KB DEAD CLEAN	30 sec.		60/30/15		
	FIGURE 8 TO A HOLD	30 sec.		60/30/15		
	PUSH-UP	30 sec.		60/30/15		
	PLANK	30 sec.		60/30/15		

		work time	KB size	rest time	reps	
Round 2	LONG CYCLE JERK	90 sec.		45 sec.	L:	R:
	SNATCH	90 sec.		45 sec.	L:	R:
	HAND 2 HAND SUMO DEADLIFT	30 sec.		60/30/15		
	SIDE BEND (LEFT AND RIGHT)	30 sec.		60/30/15		
	ALTERNATING CLEAN (DIP & SWITCH)	30 sec.		60/30/15		
	FIGURE 8 TO A HOLD	30 sec.		60/30/15		
	CLOSE GRIP PUSH-UP (MILITARY)	30 sec.		60/30/15		

		work time	KB size	rest time	reps	
Round 3	PUSH PRESS	90 sec.		45 sec.	L:	R:
	1/2 SNATCH	90 sec.		45 sec.	L:	R:
	BEHIND THE NECK SQUAT	30 sec.		60/30/15		
	WINDMILL (LEFT AND RIGHT)	30 sec.		60/30/15		
	DOUBLE KB LONG CYCLE CLEAN	30 sec.		60/30/15		
	STAGGERED PUSH-UP (EXPLOSIVE)	30 sec.		60/30/15		
	HIGH PLANK	30 sec.		60/30/15		

heart rate	comments:
start:	
end:	
5 min. post:	

Im Athletic 6 Month Workout Plan

DATE: _____

MONTH: 4
WEEK: 4
DAY: 2

WARM UP: CHOOSE ONE WARM FROM THE DYNAMIC FLOW DRILL LIST

Round 1

	work time	KB size	rest time	reps	
LONG CYCLE PRESS	90 sec.		45 sec.	L:	R:
SNATCH	90 sec.		45 sec.	L:	R:
DOUBLE SQUAT	30 sec.		60/30/15		
BARBELL GET-UP SIT-UP	30 sec.		60/30/15		
DOUBLE KB DEAD CLEAN	30 sec.		60/30/15		
FIGURE 8 TO A HOLD	30 sec.		60/30/15		
PUSH-UP	30 sec.		60/30/15		
PLANK	30 sec.		60/30/15		

Round 2

	work time	KB size	rest time	reps	
LONG CYCLE JERK	90 sec.		45 sec.	L:	R:
SNATCH	90 sec.		45 sec.	L:	R:
HAND 2 HAND SUMO DEADLIFT	30 sec.		60/30/15		
SIDE BEND (LEFT AND RIGHT)	30 sec.		60/30/15		
ALTERNATING CLEAN (DIP & SWITCH)	30 sec.		60/30/15		
FIGURE 8 TO A HOLD	30 sec.		60/30/15		
CLOSE GRIP PUSH-UP (MILITARY)	30 sec.		60/30/15		

Round 3

	work time	KB size	rest time	reps	
PUSH PRESS	90 sec.		45 sec.	L:	R:
1/2 SNATCH	90 sec.		45 sec.	L:	R:
BEHIND THE NECK SQUAT	30 sec.		60/30/15		
WINDMILL (LEFT AND RIGHT)	30 sec.		60/30/15		
DOUBLE KB LONG CYCLE CLEAN	30 sec.		60/30/15		
STAGGERED PUSH-UP (EXPLOSIVE)	30 sec.		60/30/15		
HIGH PLANK	30 sec.		60/30/15		

heart rate	comments:
start:	
end:	
5 min. post:	

Im Athletic 6 Month Workout Plan

DATE: _____

MONTH: 4
WEEK: 4
DAY: 3

WARM UP: CHOOSE ONE WARM FROM THE DYNAMIC FLOW DRILL LIST

		work time	KB size	rest time	reps	
Round 1	LONG CYCLE PRESS	90 sec.		45 sec.	L:	R:
	SNATCH	90 sec.		45 sec.	L:	R:
	DOUBLE SQUAT	30 sec.		60/30/15		
	BARBELL GET-UP SIT-UP	30 sec.		60/30/15		
	DOUBLE KB DEAD CLEAN	30 sec.		60/30/15		
	FIGURE 8 TO A HOLD	30 sec.		60/30/15		
	PUSH-UP	30 sec.		60/30/15		
	PLANK	30 sec.		60/30/15		

		work time	KB size	rest time	reps	
Round 2	LONG CYCLE JERK	90 sec.		45 sec.	L:	R:
	SNATCH	90 sec.		45 sec.	L:	R:
	HAND 2 HAND SUMO DEADLIFT	30 sec.		60/30/15		
	SIDE BEND (LEFT AND RIGHT)	30 sec.		60/30/15		
	ALTERNATING CLEAN (DIP & SWITCH)	30 sec.		60/30/15		
	FIGURE 8 TO A HOLD	30 sec.		60/30/15		
	CLOSE GRIP PUSH-UP (MILITARY)	30 sec.		60/30/15		

		work time	KB size	rest time	reps	
Round 3	PUSH PRESS	90 sec.		45 sec.	L:	R:
	1/2 SNATCH	90 sec.		45 sec.	L:	R:
	BEHIND THE NECK SQUAT	30 sec.		60/30/15		
	WINDMILL (LEFT AND RIGHT)	30 sec.		60/30/15		
	DOUBLE KB LONG CYCLE CLEAN	30 sec.		60/30/15		
	STAGGERED PUSH-UP (EXPLOSIVE)	30 sec.		60/30/15		
	HIGH PLANK	30 sec.		60/30/15		

heart rate	comments:
start:	
end:	
5 min. post:	

Im Athletic 6 Month Workout Plan

DATE: _____

MONTH: 4
WEEK: 4
DAY: 4

WARM UP: CHOOSE ONE WARM FROM THE DYNAMIC FLOW DRILL LIST

Round 1		work time	KB size	rest time	reps	
	LONG CYCLE PRESS	90 sec.		45 sec.	L:	R:
	SNATCH	90 sec.		45 sec.	L:	R:
	DOUBLE SQUAT	30 sec.		60/30/15		
	BARBELL GET-UP SIT-UP	30 sec.		60/30/15		
	DOUBLE KB DEAD CLEAN	30 sec.		60/30/15		
	FIGURE 8 TO A HOLD	30 sec.		60/30/15		
	PUSH-UP	30 sec.		60/30/15		
	PLANK	30 sec.		60/30/15		

Round 2		work time	KB size	rest time	reps	
	LONG CYCLE JERK	90 sec.		45 sec.	L:	R:
	SNATCH	90 sec.		45 sec.	L:	R:
	HAND 2 HAND SUMO DEADLIFT	30 sec.		60/30/15		
	SIDE BEND (LEFT AND RIGHT)	30 sec.		60/30/15		
	ALTERNATING CLEAN (DIP & SWITCH)	30 sec.		60/30/15		
	FIGURE 8 TO A HOLD	30 sec.		60/30/15		
	CLOSE GRIP PUSH-UP (MILITARY)	30 sec.		60/30/15		

Round 3		work time	KB size	rest time	reps	
	PUSH PRESS	90 sec.		45 sec.	L:	R:
	1/2 SNATCH	90 sec.		45 sec.	L:	R:
	BEHIND THE NECK SQUAT	30 sec.		60/30/15		
	WINDMILL (LEFT AND RIGHT)	30 sec.		60/30/15		
	DOUBLE KB LONG CYCLE CLEAN	30 sec.		60/30/15		
	STAGGERED PUSH-UP (EXPLOSIVE)	30 sec.		60/30/15		
	HIGH PLANK	30 sec.		60/30/15		

heart rate	comments:
start:	
end:	
5 min. post:	

You've finished month 4!

Benefit No. 2 to Kettlebell training:

Displaced Center of Gravity: The kettlebell's center of gravity is 6-8 inches below the center of your hand. Barbells and dumbbells center the weight with your hand. This center displacement, combined with the type of routines, incorporates more core strength into your workout. Kettlebells can do what dumbbells can do, better in fact, but not vice-versa.

Im Athletic 6 Month Workout Plan

DATE: _____

WARM UP: CHOOSE ONE WARM FROM THE DYNAMIC FLOW DRILL LIST

Round 1		work time	KB size	rest time	reps	
	JERK	120 sec.		120 sec.	L:	R:
	SNATCH	120 sec.		120 sec.	L:	R:
	DOUBLE SQUAT	30 sec.		60/30/15		
	BARBELL GET-UP SIT-UP	30 sec.		60/30/15		
	DOUBLE KB DEAD CLEAN	30 sec.		60/30/15		
	FIGURE 8 TO A HOLD	30 sec.		60/30/15		
	PUSH-UP	30 sec.		60/30/15		
	PLANK	30 sec.		60/30/15		

Round 2		work time	KB size	rest time	reps	
	LONG CYCLE JERK	120 sec.		120 sec.	L:	R:
	1/2 SNATCH	120 sec.		120 sec.	L:	R:
	HAND 2 HAND SUMO DEADLIFT	30 sec.		60/30/15		
	SIDE BEND (LEFT AND RIGHT)	30 sec.		60/30/15		
	ALTERNATING CLEAN (DIP & SWITCH)	30 sec.		60/30/15		
	FIGURE 8 TO A HOLD	30 sec.		60/30/15		
	CLOSE GRIP PUSH-UP (MILITARY)	30 sec.		60/30/15		

Round 3		work time	KB size	rest time	reps	
	LONG CYCLE PRESS	120 sec.		120 sec.	L:	R:
	1/2 SNATCH	120 sec.		120 sec.	L:	R:
	BEHIND THE NECK SQUAT	30 sec.		60/30/15		
	WINDMILL (LEFT AND RIGHT)	30 sec.		60/30/15		
	DOUBLE KB LONG CYCLE CLEAN	30 sec.		60/30/15		
	STAGGERED PUSH-UP (EXPLOSIVE)	30 sec.		60/30/15		
	HIGH PLANK	30 sec.		60/30/15		

heart rate	comments:
start:	
end:	
5 min. post:	

Im Athletic 6 Month Workout Plan

DATE: _____

MONTH: 5
WEEK: 1
DAY: 2

WARM UP: CHOOSE ONE WARM FROM THE DYNAMIC FLOW DRILL LIST

		work time	KB size	rest time	reps	
Round 1	JERK	120 sec.		120 sec.	L:	R:
	SNATCH	120 sec.		120 sec.	L:	R:
	DOUBLE SQUAT	30 sec.		60/30/15		
	BARBELL GET-UP SIT-UP	30 sec.		60/30/15		
	DOUBLE KB DEAD CLEAN	30 sec.		60/30/15		
	FIGURE 8 TO A HOLD	30 sec.		60/30/15		
	PUSH-UP	30 sec.		60/30/15		
	PLANK	30 sec.		60/30/15		

		work time	KB size	rest time	reps	
Round 2	LONG CYCLE JERK	120 sec.		120 sec.	L:	R:
	1/2 SNATCH	120 sec.		120 sec.	L:	R:
	HAND 2 HAND SUMO DEADLIFT	30 sec.		60/30/15		
	SIDE BEND (LEFT AND RIGHT)	30 sec.		60/30/15		
	ALTERNATING CLEAN (DIP & SWITCH)	30 sec.		60/30/15		
	FIGURE 8 TO A HOLD	30 sec.		60/30/15		
	CLOSE GRIP PUSH-UP (MILITARY)	30 sec.		60/30/15		

		work time	KB size	rest time	reps	
Round 3	LONG CYCLE PRESS	120 sec.		120 sec.	L:	R:
	1/2 SNATCH	120 sec.		120 sec.	L:	R:
	BEHIND THE NECK SQUAT	30 sec.		60/30/15		
	WINDMILL (LEFT AND RIGHT)	30 sec.		60/30/15		
	DOUBLE KB LONG CYCLE CLEAN	30 sec.		60/30/15		
	STAGGERED PUSH-UP (EXPLOSIVE)	30 sec.		60/30/15		
	HIGH PLANK	30 sec.		60/30/15		

heart rate	comments:
start:	
end:	
5 min. post:	

Im Athletic 6 Month Workout Plan

DATE: _____

MONTH: 5
WEEK: 1
DAY: 3

WARM UP: CHOOSE ONE WARM FROM THE DYNAMIC FLOW DRILL LIST

Round 1

	work time	KB size	rest time	reps	
JERK	120 sec.		120 sec.	L:	R:
SNATCH	120 sec.		120 sec.	L:	R:
DOUBLE SQUAT	30 sec.		60/30/15		
BARBELL GET-UP SIT-UP	30 sec.		60/30/15		
DOUBLE KB DEAD CLEAN	30 sec.		60/30/15		
FIGURE 8 TO A HOLD	30 sec.		60/30/15		
PUSH-UP	30 sec.		60/30/15		
PLANK	30 sec.		60/30/15		

Round 2

	work time	KB size	rest time	reps	
LONG CYCLE JERK	120 sec.		120 sec.	L:	R:
1/2 SNATCH	120 sec.		120 sec.	L:	R:
HAND 2 HAND SUMO DEADLIFT	30 sec.		60/30/15		
SIDE BEND (LEFT AND RIGHT)	30 sec.		60/30/15		
ALTERNATING CLEAN (DIP & SWITCH)	30 sec.		60/30/15		
FIGURE 8 TO A HOLD	30 sec.		60/30/15		
CLOSE GRIP PUSH-UP (MILITARY)	30 sec.		60/30/15		

Round 3

	work time	KB size	rest time	reps	
LONG CYCLE PRESS	120 sec.		120 sec.	L:	R:
1/2 SNATCH	120 sec.		120 sec.	L:	R:
BEHIND THE NECK SQUAT	30 sec.		60/30/15		
WINDMILL (LEFT AND RIGHT)	30 sec.		60/30/15		
DOUBLE KB LONG CYCLE CLEAN	30 sec.		60/30/15		
STAGGERED PUSH-UP (EXPLOSIVE)	30 sec.		60/30/15		
HIGH PLANK	30 sec.		60/30/15		

heart rate	comments:
start:	
end:	
5 min. post:	

Im Athletic 6 Month Workout Plan

DATE: _____

WARM UP: CHOOSE ONE WARM FROM THE DYNAMIC FLOW DRILL LIST

		work time	KB size	rest time	reps	
Round 1	JERK	120 sec.		120 sec.	L:	R:
	SNATCH	120 sec.		120 sec.	L:	R:
	DOUBLE SQUAT	30 sec.		60/30/15		
	BARBELL GET-UP SIT-UP	30 sec.		60/30/15		
	DOUBLE KB DEAD CLEAN	30 sec.		60/30/15		
	FIGURE 8 TO A HOLD	30 sec.		60/30/15		
	PUSH-UP	30 sec.		60/30/15		
	PLANK	30 sec.		60/30/15		

		work time	KB size	rest time	reps	
Round 2	LONG CYCLE JERK	120 sec.		120 sec.	L:	R:
	1/2 SNATCH	120 sec.		120 sec.	L:	R:
	HAND 2 HAND SUMO DEADLIFT	30 sec.		60/30/15		
	SIDE BEND (LEFT AND RIGHT)	30 sec.		60/30/15		
	ALTERNATING CLEAN (DIP & SWITCH)	30 sec.		60/30/15		
	FIGURE 8 TO A HOLD	30 sec.		60/30/15		
	CLOSE GRIP PUSH-UP (MILITARY)	30 sec.		60/30/15		

		work time	KB size	rest time	reps	
Round 3	LONG CYCLE PRESS	120 sec.		120 sec.	L:	R:
	1/2 SNATCH	120 sec.		120 sec.	L:	R:
	BEHIND THE NECK SQUAT	30 sec.		60/30/15		
	WINDMILL (LEFT AND RIGHT)	30 sec.		60/30/15		
	DOUBLE KB LONG CYCLE CLEAN	30 sec.		60/30/15		
	STAGGERED PUSH-UP (EXPLOSIVE)	30 sec.		60/30/15		
	HIGH PLANK	30 sec.		60/30/15		

heart rate	comments:
start:	
end:	
5 min. post:	

Im Athletic 6 Month Workout Plan

DATE: _____

MONTH: 5
WEEK: 2
DAY: 1

WARM UP: CHOOSE ONE WARM FROM THE DYNAMIC FLOW DRILL LIST

Round 1

	work time	KB size	rest time	reps	
JERK	120 sec.		90 sec.	L:	R:
SNATCH	120 sec.		90 sec.	L:	R:
DOUBLE SQUAT	30 sec.		60/30/15		
BARBELL GET-UP SIT-UP	30 sec.		60/30/15		
DOUBLE KB DEAD CLEAN	30 sec.		60/30/15		
FIGURE 8 TO A HOLD	30 sec.		60/30/15		
PUSH-UP	30 sec.		60/30/15		
PLANK	30 sec.		60/30/15		

Round 2

	work time	KB size	rest time	reps	
JERK	120 sec.		90 sec.	L:	R:
1/2 SNATCH	120 sec.		90 sec.	L:	R:
HAND 2 HAND SUMO DEADLIFT	30 sec.		60/30/15		
SIDE BEND (LEFT AND RIGHT)	30 sec.		60/30/15		
ALTERNATING CLEAN (DIP & SWITCH)	30 sec.		60/30/15		
FIGURE 8 TO A HOLD	30 sec.		60/30/15		
CLOSE GRIP PUSH-UP (MILITARY)	30 sec.		60/30/15		

Round 3

	work time	KB size	rest time	reps	
LONG CYCLE JERK	120 sec.		90 sec.	L:	R:
SNATCH	120 sec.		90 sec.	L:	R:
BEHIND THE NECK SQUAT	30 sec.		60/30/15		
WINDMILL (LEFT AND RIGHT)	30 sec.		60/30/15		
DOUBLE KB LONG CYCLE CLEAN	30 sec.		60/30/15		
STAGGERED PUSH-UP (EXPLOSIVE)	30 sec.		60/30/15		
HIGH PLANK	30 sec.		60/30/15		

heart rate	comments:
start:	
end:	
5 min. post:	

Im Athletic 6 Month Workout Plan

DATE: _____

MONTH: 5
WEEK: 2
DAY: 2

WARM UP: CHOOSE ONE WARM FROM THE DYNAMIC FLOW DRILL LIST

Round 1		work time	KB size	rest time	reps	
	JERK	120 sec.		90 sec.	L:	R:
	SNATCH	120 sec.		90 sec.	L:	R:
	DOUBLE SQUAT	30 sec.		60/30/15		
	BARBELL GET-UP SIT-UP	30 sec.		60/30/15		
	DOUBLE KB DEAD CLEAN	30 sec.		60/30/15		
	FIGURE 8 TO A HOLD	30 sec.		60/30/15		
	PUSH-UP	30 sec.		60/30/15		
	PLANK	30 sec.		60/30/15		

Round 2		work time	KB size	rest time	reps	
	JERK	120 sec.		90 sec.	L:	R:
	1/2 SNATCH	120 sec.		90 sec.	L:	R:
	HAND 2 HAND SUMO DEADLIFT	30 sec.		60/30/15		
	SIDE BEND (LEFT AND RIGHT)	30 sec.		60/30/15		
	ALTERNATING CLEAN (DIP & SWITCH)	30 sec.		60/30/15		
	FIGURE 8 TO A HOLD	30 sec.		60/30/15		
	CLOSE GRIP PUSH-UP (MILITARY)	30 sec.		60/30/15		

Round 3		work time	KB size	rest time	reps	
	LONG CYCLE JERK	120 sec.		90 sec.	L:	R:
	SNATCH	120 sec.		90 sec.	L:	R:
	BEHIND THE NECK SQUAT	30 sec.		60/30/15		
	WINDMILL (LEFT AND RIGHT)	30 sec.		60/30/15		
	DOUBLE KB LONG CYCLE CLEAN	30 sec.		60/30/15		
	STAGGERED PUSH-UP (EXPLOSIVE)	30 sec.		60/30/15		
	HIGH PLANK	30 sec.		60/30/15		

heart rate	comments:
start:	
end:	
5 min. post:	

Im Athletic 6 Month Workout Plan

DATE: _____

WARM UP: CHOOSE ONE WARM FROM THE DYNAMIC FLOW DRILL LIST

		work time	KB size	rest time	reps	
Round 1	JERK	120 sec.		90 sec.	L:	R:
	SNATCH	120 sec.		90 sec.	L:	R:
	DOUBLE SQUAT	30 sec.		60/30/15		
	BARBELL GET-UP SIT-UP	30 sec.		60/30/15		
	DOUBLE KB DEAD CLEAN	30 sec.		60/30/15		
	FIGURE 8 TO A HOLD	30 sec.		60/30/15		
	PUSH-UP	30 sec.		60/30/15		
	PLANK	30 sec.		60/30/15		

		work time	KB size	rest time	reps	
Round 2	JERK	120 sec.		90 sec.	L:	R:
	1/2 SNATCH	120 sec.		90 sec.	L:	R:
	HAND 2 HAND SUMO DEADLIFT	30 sec.		60/30/15		
	SIDE BEND (LEFT AND RIGHT)	30 sec.		60/30/15		
	ALTERNATING CLEAN (DIP & SWITCH)	30 sec.		60/30/15		
	FIGURE 8 TO A HOLD	30 sec.		60/30/15		
	CLOSE GRIP PUSH-UP (MILITARY)	30 sec.		60/30/15		

		work time	KB size	rest time	reps	
Round 3	LONG CYCLE JERK	120 sec.		90 sec.	L:	R:
	SNATCH	120 sec.		90 sec.	L:	R:
	BEHIND THE NECK SQUAT	30 sec.		60/30/15		
	WINDMILL (LEFT AND RIGHT)	30 sec.		60/30/15		
	DOUBLE KB LONG CYCLE CLEAN	30 sec.		60/30/15		
	STAGGERED PUSH-UP (EXPLOSIVE)	30 sec.		60/30/15		
	HIGH PLANK	30 sec.		60/30/15		

heart rate	comments:
start:	
end:	
5 min. post:	

Im Athletic 6 Month Workout Plan

DATE: _____

MONTH: 5
WEEK: 2
DAY: 4

WARM UP: CHOOSE ONE WARM FROM THE DYNAMIC FLOW DRILL LIST

		work time	KB size	rest time	reps	
Round 1	JERK	120 sec.		90 sec.	L:	R:
	SNATCH	120 sec.		90 sec.	L:	R:
	DOUBLE SQUAT	30 sec.		60/30/15		
	BARBELL GET-UP SIT-UP	30 sec.		60/30/15		
	DOUBLE KB DEAD CLEAN	30 sec.		60/30/15		
	FIGURE 8 TO A HOLD	30 sec.		60/30/15		
	PUSH-UP	30 sec.		60/30/15		
	PLANK	30 sec.		60/30/15		

		work time	KB size	rest time	reps	
Round 2	JERK	120 sec.		90 sec.	L:	R:
	1/2 SNATCH	120 sec.		90 sec.	L:	R:
	HAND 2 HAND SUMO DEADLIFT	30 sec.		60/30/15		
	SIDE BEND (LEFT AND RIGHT)	30 sec.		60/30/15		
	ALTERNATING CLEAN (DIP & SWITCH)	30 sec.		60/30/15		
	FIGURE 8 TO A HOLD	30 sec.		60/30/15		
	CLOSE GRIP PUSH-UP (MILITARY)	30 sec.		60/30/15		

		work time	KB size	rest time	reps	
Round 3	LONG CYCLE JERK	120 sec.		90 sec.	L:	R:
	SNATCH	120 sec.		90 sec.	L:	R:
	BEHIND THE NECK SQUAT	30 sec.		60/30/15		
	WINDMILL (LEFT AND RIGHT)	30 sec.		60/30/15		
	DOUBLE KB LONG CYCLE CLEAN	30 sec.		60/30/15		
	STAGGERED PUSH-UP (EXPLOSIVE)	30 sec.		60/30/15		
	HIGH PLANK	30 sec.		60/30/15		

heart rate	comments:
start:	
end:	
5 min. post:	

Im Athletic 6 Month Workout Plan

DATE: _____

WARM UP: CHOOSE ONE WARM FROM THE DYNAMIC FLOW DRILL LIST

		work time	KB size	rest time	reps	
Round 1	BOTTOM UP JERK	120 sec.		60 sec.	L:	R:
	SNATCH	120 sec.		60 sec.	L:	R:
	DOUBLE SQUAT	30 sec.		60/30/15		
	BARBELL GET-UP SIT-UP	30 sec.		60/30/15		
	DOUBLE KB DEAD CLEAN	30 sec.		60/30/15		
	FIGURE 8 TO A HOLD	30 sec.		60/30/15		
	PUSH-UP	30 sec.		60/30/15		
	PLANK	30 sec.		60/30/15		

		work time	KB size	rest time	reps	
Round 2	LONG CYCLE JERK	120 sec.		60 sec.	L:	R:
	1/2 SNATCH	120 sec.		60 sec.	L:	R:
	HAND 2 HAND SUMO DEADLIFT	30 sec.		60/30/15		
	SIDE BEND (LEFT AND RIGHT)	30 sec.		60/30/15		
	ALTERNATING CLEAN (DIP & SWITCH)	30 sec.		60/30/15		
	FIGURE 8 TO A HOLD	30 sec.		60/30/15		
	CLOSE GRIP PUSH-UP (MILITARY)	30 sec.		60/30/15		

		work time	KB size	rest time	reps	
Round 3	PRESS	120 sec.		60 sec.	L:	R:
	SNATCH	120 sec.		60 sec.	L:	R:
	BEHIND THE NECK SQUAT	30 sec.		60/30/15		
	WINDMILL (LEFT AND RIGHT)	30 sec.		60/30/15		
	DOUBLE KB LONG CYCLE CLEAN	30 sec.		60/30/15		
	STAGGERED PUSH-UP (EXPLOSIVE)	30 sec.		60/30/15		
	HIGH PLANK	30 sec.		60/30/15		

heart rate	comments:
start:	
end:	
5 min. post:	

Im Athletic 6 Month Workout Plan

DATE: _____

WARM UP: CHOOSE ONE WARM FROM THE DYNAMIC FLOW DRILL LIST

		work time	KB size	rest time	reps	
Round 1	BOTTOM UP JERK	120 sec.		60 sec.	L:	R:
	SNATCH	120 sec.		60 sec.	L:	R:
	DOUBLE SQUAT	30 sec.		60/30/15		
	BARBELL GET-UP SIT-UP	30 sec.		60/30/15		
	DOUBLE KB DEAD CLEAN	30 sec.		60/30/15		
	FIGURE 8 TO A HOLD	30 sec.		60/30/15		
	PUSH-UP	30 sec.		60/30/15		
	PLANK	30 sec.		60/30/15		

		work time	KB size	rest time	reps	
Round 2	LONG CYCLE JERK	120 sec.		60 sec.	L:	R:
	1/2 SNATCH	120 sec.		60 sec.	L:	R:
	HAND 2 HAND SUMO DEADLIFT	30 sec.		60/30/15		
	SIDE BEND (LEFT AND RIGHT)	30 sec.		60/30/15		
	ALTERNATING CLEAN (DIP & SWITCH)	30 sec.		60/30/15		
	FIGURE 8 TO A HOLD	30 sec.		60/30/15		
	CLOSE GRIP PUSH-UP (MILITARY)	30 sec.		60/30/15		

		work time	KB size	rest time	reps	
Round 3	PRESS	120 sec.		60 sec.	L:	R:
	SNATCH	120 sec.		60 sec.	L:	R:
	BEHIND THE NECK SQUAT	30 sec.		60/30/15		
	WINDMILL (LEFT AND RIGHT)	30 sec.		60/30/15		
	DOUBLE KB LONG CYCLE CLEAN	30 sec.		60/30/15		
	STAGGERED PUSH-UP (EXPLOSIVE)	30 sec.		60/30/15		
	HIGH PLANK	30 sec.		60/30/15		

heart rate	comments:
start:	
end:	
5 min. post:	

Im Athletic 6 Month Workout Plan

DATE: _____

WARM UP: CHOOSE ONE WARM FROM THE DYNAMIC FLOW DRILL LIST

Round 1		work time	KB size	rest time	reps	
	BOTTOM UP JERK	120 sec.		60 sec.	L:	R:
	SNATCH	120 sec.		60 sec.	L:	R:
	DOUBLE SQUAT	30 sec.		60/30/15		
	BARBELL GET-UP SIT-UP	30 sec.		60/30/15		
	DOUBLE KB DEAD CLEAN	30 sec.		60/30/15		
	FIGURE 8 TO A HOLD	30 sec.		60/30/15		
	PUSH-UP	30 sec.		60/30/15		
	PLANK	30 sec.		60/30/15		

Round 2		work time	KB size	rest time	reps	
	LONG CYCLE JERK	120 sec.		60 sec.	L:	R:
	1/2 SNATCH	120 sec.		60 sec.	L:	R:
	HAND 2 HAND SUMO DEADLIFT	30 sec.		60/30/15		
	SIDE BEND (LEFT AND RIGHT)	30 sec.		60/30/15		
	ALTERNATING CLEAN (DIP & SWITCH)	30 sec.		60/30/15		
	FIGURE 8 TO A HOLD	30 sec.		60/30/15		
	CLOSE GRIP PUSH-UP (MILITARY)	30 sec.		60/30/15		

Round 3		work time	KB size	rest time	reps	
	PRESS	120 sec.		60 sec.	L:	R:
	SNATCH	120 sec.		60 sec.	L:	R:
	BEHIND THE NECK SQUAT	30 sec.		60/30/15		
	WINDMILL (LEFT AND RIGHT)	30 sec.		60/30/15		
	DOUBLE KB LONG CYCLE CLEAN	30 sec.		60/30/15		
	STAGGERED PUSH-UP (EXPLOSIVE)	30 sec.		60/30/15		
	HIGH PLANK	30 sec.		60/30/15		

heart rate	comments:
start:	
end:	
5 min. post:	

Im Athletic 6 Month Workout Plan

DATE: _____

WARM UP: CHOOSE ONE WARM FROM THE DYNAMIC FLOW DRILL LIST

		work time	KB size	rest time	reps	
Round 1	BOTTOM UP JERK	120 sec.		60 sec.	L:	R:
	SNATCH	120 sec.		60 sec.	L:	R:
	DOUBLE SQUAT	30 sec.		60/30/15		
	BARBELL GET-UP SIT-UP	30 sec.		60/30/15		
	DOUBLE KB DEAD CLEAN	30 sec.		60/30/15		
	FIGURE 8 TO A HOLD	30 sec.		60/30/15		
	PUSH-UP	30 sec.		60/30/15		
	PLANK	30 sec.		60/30/15		

		work time	KB size	rest time	reps	
Round 2	LONG CYCLE JERK	120 sec.		60 sec.	L:	R:
	1/2 SNATCH	120 sec.		60 sec.	L:	R:
	HAND 2 HAND SUMO DEADLIFT	30 sec.		60/30/15		
	SIDE BEND (LEFT AND RIGHT)	30 sec.		60/30/15		
	ALTERNATING CLEAN (DIP & SWITCH)	30 sec.		60/30/15		
	FIGURE 8 TO A HOLD	30 sec.		60/30/15		
	CLOSE GRIP PUSH-UP (MILITARY)	30 sec.		60/30/15		

		work time	KB size	rest time	reps	
Round 3	PRESS	120 sec.		60 sec.	L:	R:
	SNATCH	120 sec.		60 sec.	L:	R:
	BEHIND THE NECK SQUAT	30 sec.		60/30/15		
	WINDMILL (LEFT AND RIGHT)	30 sec.		60/30/15		
	DOUBLE KB LONG CYCLE CLEAN	30 sec.		60/30/15		
	STAGGERED PUSH-UP (EXPLOSIVE)	30 sec.		60/30/15		
	HIGH PLANK	30 sec.		60/30/15		

heart rate	comments:
start:	
end:	
5 min. post:	

Im Athletic 6 Month Workout Plan

DATE: _____

WARM UP: CHOOSE ONE WARM FROM THE DYNAMIC FLOW DRILL LIST

		work time	KB size	rest time	reps	
Round 1	LONG CYCLE BOTTOM UP PRESS	120 sec.		30 sec.	L:	R:
	SNATCH	120 sec.		30 sec.	L:	R:
	DOUBLE SQUAT	30 sec.		60/30/15		
	BARBELL GET-UP SIT-UP	30 sec.		60/30/15		
	DOUBLE KB DEAD CLEAN	30 sec.		60/30/15		
	FIGURE 8 TO A HOLD	30 sec.		60/30/15		
	PUSH-UP	30 sec.		60/30/15		
	PLANK	30 sec.		60/30/15		

		work time	KB size	rest time	reps	
Round 2	PUSH PRESS	120 sec.		30 sec.	L:	R:
	SNATCH	120 sec.		30 sec.	L:	R:
	HAND 2 HAND SUMO DEADLIFT	30 sec.		60/30/15		
	SIDE BEND (LEFT AND RIGHT)	30 sec.		60/30/15		
	ALTERNATING CLEAN (DIP & SWITCH)	30 sec.		60/30/15		
	FIGURE 8 TO A HOLD	30 sec.		60/30/15		
	CLOSE GRIP PUSH-UP (MILITARY)	30 sec.		60/30/15		

		work time	KB size	rest time	reps	
Round 3	LONG CYCLE JERK	120 sec.		30 sec.	L:	R:
	SNATCH	120 sec.		30 sec.	L:	R:
	BEHIND THE NECK SQUAT	30 sec.		60/30/15		
	WINDMILL (LEFT AND RIGHT)	30 sec.		60/30/15		
	DOUBLE KB LONG CYCLE CLEAN	30 sec.		60/30/15		
	STAGGERED PUSH-UP (EXPLOSIVE)	30 sec.		60/30/15		
	HIGH PLANK	30 sec.		60/30/15		

heart rate	comments:
start:	
end:	
5 min. post:	

Im Athletic 6 Month Workout Plan

DATE: _____

WARM UP: CHOOSE ONE WARM FROM THE DYNAMIC FLOW DRILL LIST

		work time	KB size	rest time	reps	
Round 1	LONG CYCLE BOTTOM UP PRESS	120 sec.		30 sec.	L:	R:
	SNATCH	120 sec.		30 sec.	L:	R:
	DOUBLE SQUAT	30 sec.		60/30/15		
	BARBELL GET-UP SIT-UP	30 sec.		60/30/15		
	DOUBLE KB DEAD CLEAN	30 sec.		60/30/15		
	FIGURE 8 TO A HOLD	30 sec.		60/30/15		
	PUSH-UP	30 sec.		60/30/15		
	PLANK	30 sec.		60/30/15		

		work time	KB size	rest time	reps	
Round 2	PUSH PRESS	120 sec.		30 sec.	L:	R:
	SNATCH	120 sec.		30 sec.	L:	R:
	HAND 2 HAND SUMO DEADLIFT	30 sec.		60/30/15		
	SIDE BEND (LEFT AND RIGHT)	30 sec.		60/30/15		
	ALTERNATING CLEAN (DIP & SWITCH)	30 sec.		60/30/15		
	FIGURE 8 TO A HOLD	30 sec.		60/30/15		
	CLOSE GRIP PUSH-UP (MILITARY)	30 sec.		60/30/15		

		work time	KB size	rest time	reps	
Round 3	LONG CYCLE JERK	120 sec.		30 sec.	L:	R:
	SNATCH	120 sec.		30 sec.	L:	R:
	BEHIND THE NECK SQUAT	30 sec.		60/30/15		
	WINDMILL (LEFT AND RIGHT)	30 sec.		60/30/15		
	DOUBLE KB LONG CYCLE CLEAN	30 sec.		60/30/15		
	STAGGERED PUSH-UP (EXPLOSIVE)	30 sec.		60/30/15		
	HIGH PLANK	30 sec.		60/30/15		

heart rate	comments:
start:	
end:	
5 min. post:	

Im Athletic 6 Month Workout Plan

DATE: _____

WARM UP: CHOOSE ONE WARM FROM THE DYNAMIC FLOW DRILL LIST

		work time	KB size	rest time	reps	
Round 1	LONG CYCLE BOTTOM UP PRESS	120 sec.		30 sec.	L:	R:
	SNATCH	120 sec.		30 sec.	L:	R:
	DOUBLE SQUAT	30 sec.		60/30/15		
	BARBELL GET-UP SIT-UP	30 sec.		60/30/15		
	DOUBLE KB DEAD CLEAN	30 sec.		60/30/15		
	FIGURE 8 TO A HOLD	30 sec.		60/30/15		
	PUSH-UP	30 sec.		60/30/15		
	PLANK	30 sec.		60/30/15		

		work time	KB size	rest time	reps	
Round 2	PUSH PRESS	120 sec.		30 sec.	L:	R:
	SNATCH	120 sec.		30 sec.	L:	R:
	HAND 2 HAND SUMO DEADLIFT	30 sec.		60/30/15		
	SIDE BEND (LEFT AND RIGHT)	30 sec.		60/30/15		
	ALTERNATING CLEAN (DIP & SWITCH)	30 sec.		60/30/15		
	FIGURE 8 TO A HOLD	30 sec.		60/30/15		
	CLOSE GRIP PUSH-UP (MILITARY)	30 sec.		60/30/15		

		work time	KB size	rest time	reps	
Round 3	LONG CYCLE JERK	120 sec.		30 sec.	L:	R:
	SNATCH	120 sec.		30 sec.	L:	R:
	BEHIND THE NECK SQUAT	30 sec.		60/30/15		
	WINDMILL (LEFT AND RIGHT)	30 sec.		60/30/15		
	DOUBLE KB LONG CYCLE CLEAN	30 sec.		60/30/15		
	STAGGERED PUSH-UP (EXPLOSIVE)	30 sec.		60/30/15		
	HIGH PLANK	30 sec.		60/30/15		

heart rate	comments:
start:	
end:	
5 min. post:	

Im Athletic 6 Month Workout Plan

DATE: _____

WARM UP: CHOOSE ONE WARM FROM THE DYNAMIC FLOW DRILL LIST

		work time	KB size	rest time	reps	
Round 1	LONG CYCLE BOTTOM UP PRESS	120 sec.		30 sec.	L:	R:
	SNATCH	120 sec.		30 sec.	L:	R:
	DOUBLE SQUAT	30 sec.		60/30/15		
	BARBELL GET-UP SIT-UP	30 sec.		60/30/15		
	DOUBLE KB DEAD CLEAN	30 sec.		60/30/15		
	FIGURE 8 TO A HOLD	30 sec.		60/30/15		
	PUSH-UP	30 sec.		60/30/15		
	PLANK	30 sec.		60/30/15		

		work time	KB size	rest time	reps	
Round 2	PUSH PRESS	120 sec.		30 sec.	L:	R:
	SNATCH	120 sec.		30 sec.	L:	R:
	HAND 2 HAND SUMO DEADLIFT	30 sec.		60/30/15		
	SIDE BEND (LEFT AND RIGHT)	30 sec.		60/30/15		
	ALTERNATING CLEAN (DIP & SWITCH)	30 sec.		60/30/15		
	FIGURE 8 TO A HOLD	30 sec.		60/30/15		
	CLOSE GRIP PUSH-UP (MILITARY)	30 sec.		60/30/15		

		work time	KB size	rest time	reps	
Round 3	LONG CYCLE JERK	120 sec.		30 sec.	L:	R:
	SNATCH	120 sec.		30 sec.	L:	R:
	BEHIND THE NECK SQUAT	30 sec.		60/30/15		
	WINDMILL (LEFT AND RIGHT)	30 sec.		60/30/15		
	DOUBLE KB LONG CYCLE CLEAN	30 sec.		60/30/15		
	STAGGERED PUSH-UP (EXPLOSIVE)	30 sec.		60/30/15		
	HIGH PLANK	30 sec.		60/30/15		

heart rate	comments:
start:	
end:	
5 min. post:	

You've finished month 5!

"I've got a theory that if you give 100 percent all of the time, somehow things will work out in the end." – **Larry Bird**

Im Athletic 6 Month Workout Plan

DATE: _____

WARM UP: CHOOSE ONE WARM FROM THE DYNAMIC FLOW DRILL LIST

		work time	KB size	rest time	reps	
Round 1	JERK	180 sec.		120 sec.	L:	R:
	SNATCH	180 sec.		120 sec.	L:	R:
	DOUBLE SQUAT	30 sec.		60/30/15		
	BARBELL GET-UP SIT-UP	30 sec.		60/30/15		
	DOUBLE KB DEAD CLEAN	30 sec.		60/30/15		
	FIGURE 8 TO A HOLD	30 sec.		60/30/15		
	PUSH-UP	30 sec.		60/30/15		
	PLANK	30 sec.		60/30/15		

		work time	KB size	rest time	reps	
Round 2	LONG CYCLE JERK	180 sec.		120 sec.	L:	R:
	1/2 SNATCH	180 sec.		120 sec.	L:	R:
	HAND 2 HAND SUMO DEADLIFT	30 sec.		60/30/15		
	SIDE BEND (LEFT AND RIGHT)	30 sec.		60/30/15		
	ALTERNATING CLEAN (DIP & SWITCH)	30 sec.		60/30/15		
	FIGURE 8 TO A HOLD	30 sec.		60/30/15		
	CLOSE GRIP PUSH-UP (MILITARY)	30 sec.		60/30/15		

		work time	KB size	rest time	reps	
Round 3	PRESS	180 sec.		120 sec.	L:	R:
	SNATCH	180 sec.		120 sec.	L:	R:
	BEHIND THE NECK SQUAT	30 sec.		60/30/15		
	WINDMILL (LEFT AND RIGHT)	30 sec.		60/30/15		
	DOUBLE KB LONG CYCLE CLEAN	30 sec.		60/30/15		
	STAGGERED PUSH-UP (EXPLOSIVE)	30 sec.		60/30/15		
	HIGH PLANK	30 sec.		60/30/15		

heart rate	comments:
start:	
end:	
5 min. post:	

Im Athletic 6 Month Workout Plan

DATE: _____

WARM UP: CHOOSE ONE WARM FROM THE DYNAMIC FLOW DRILL LIST

		work time	KB size	rest time	reps	
Round 1	JERK	180 sec.		120 sec.	L:	R:
	SNATCH	180 sec.		120 sec.	L:	R:
	DOUBLE SQUAT	30 sec.		60/30/15		
	BARBELL GET-UP SIT-UP	30 sec.		60/30/15		
	DOUBLE KB DEAD CLEAN	30 sec.		60/30/15		
	FIGURE 8 TO A HOLD	30 sec.		60/30/15		
	PUSH-UP	30 sec.		60/30/15		
	PLANK	30 sec.		60/30/15		

		work time	KB size	rest time	reps	
Round 2	LONG CYCLE JERK	180 sec.		120 sec.	L:	R:
	1/2 SNATCH	180 sec.		120 sec.	L:	R:
	HAND 2 HAND SUMO DEADLIFT	30 sec.		60/30/15		
	SIDE BEND (LEFT AND RIGHT)	30 sec.		60/30/15		
	ALTERNATING CLEAN (DIP & SWITCH)	30 sec.		60/30/15		
	FIGURE 8 TO A HOLD	30 sec.		60/30/15		
	CLOSE GRIP PUSH-UP (MILITARY)	30 sec.		60/30/15		

		work time	KB size	rest time	reps	
Round 3	PRESS	180 sec.		120 sec.	L:	R:
	SNATCH	180 sec.		120 sec.	L:	R:
	BEHIND THE NECK SQUAT	30 sec.		60/30/15		
	WINDMILL (LEFT AND RIGHT)	30 sec.		60/30/15		
	DOUBLE KB LONG CYCLE CLEAN	30 sec.		60/30/15		
	STAGGERED PUSH-UP (EXPLOSIVE)	30 sec.		60/30/15		
	HIGH PLANK	30 sec.		60/30/15		

heart rate	comments:
start:	
end:	
5 min. post:	

Im Athletic 6 Month Workout Plan

DATE: _____

WARM UP: CHOOSE ONE WARM FROM THE DYNAMIC FLOW DRILL LIST

		work time	KB size	rest time	reps	
Round 1	JERK	180 sec.		120 sec.	L:	R:
	SNATCH	180 sec.		120 sec.	L:	R:
	DOUBLE SQUAT	30 sec.		60/30/15		
	BARBELL GET-UP SIT-UP	30 sec.		60/30/15		
	DOUBLE KB DEAD CLEAN	30 sec.		60/30/15		
	FIGURE 8 TO A HOLD	30 sec.		60/30/15		
	PUSH-UP	30 sec.		60/30/15		
	PLANK	30 sec.		60/30/15		

		work time	KB size	rest time	reps	
Round 2	LONG CYCLE JERK	180 sec.		120 sec.	L:	R:
	1/2 SNATCH	180 sec.		120 sec.	L:	R:
	HAND 2 HAND SUMO DEADLIFT	30 sec.		60/30/15		
	SIDE BEND (LEFT AND RIGHT)	30 sec.		60/30/15		
	ALTERNATING CLEAN (DIP & SWITCH)	30 sec.		60/30/15		
	FIGURE 8 TO A HOLD	30 sec.		60/30/15		
	CLOSE GRIP PUSH-UP (MILITARY)	30 sec.		60/30/15		

		work time	KB size	rest time	reps	
Round 3	PRESS	180 sec.		120 sec.	L:	R:
	SNATCH	180 sec.		120 sec.	L:	R:
	BEHIND THE NECK SQUAT	30 sec.		60/30/15		
	WINDMILL (LEFT AND RIGHT)	30 sec.		60/30/15		
	DOUBLE KB LONG CYCLE CLEAN	30 sec.		60/30/15		
	STAGGERED PUSH-UP (EXPLOSIVE)	30 sec.		60/30/15		
	HIGH PLANK	30 sec.		60/30/15		

heart rate	comments:
start:	
end:	
5 min. post:	

Im Athletic 6 Month Workout Plan

DATE: _____

WARM UP: CHOOSE ONE WARM FROM THE DYNAMIC FLOW DRILL LIST

		work time	KB size	rest time	reps	
Round 1	JERK	180 sec.		120 sec.	L:	R:
	SNATCH	180 sec.		120 sec.	L:	R:
	DOUBLE SQUAT	30 sec.		60/30/15		
	BARBELL GET-UP SIT-UP	30 sec.		60/30/15		
	DOUBLE KB DEAD CLEAN	30 sec.		60/30/15		
	FIGURE 8 TO A HOLD	30 sec.		60/30/15		
	PUSH-UP	30 sec.		60/30/15		
	PLANK	30 sec.		60/30/15		

		work time	KB size	rest time	reps	
Round 2	LONG CYCLE JERK	180 sec.		120 sec.	L:	R:
	1/2 SNATCH	180 sec.		120 sec.	L:	R:
	HAND 2 HAND SUMO DEADLIFT	30 sec.		60/30/15		
	SIDE BEND (LEFT AND RIGHT)	30 sec.		60/30/15		
	ALTERNATING CLEAN (DIP & SWITCH)	30 sec.		60/30/15		
	FIGURE 8 TO A HOLD	30 sec.		60/30/15		
	CLOSE GRIP PUSH-UP (MILITARY)	30 sec.		60/30/15		

		work time	KB size	rest time	reps	
Round 3	PRESS	180 sec.		120 sec.	L:	R:
	SNATCH	180 sec.		120 sec.	L:	R:
	BEHIND THE NECK SQUAT	30 sec.		60/30/15		
	WINDMILL (LEFT AND RIGHT)	30 sec.		60/30/15		
	DOUBLE KB LONG CYCLE CLEAN	30 sec.		60/30/15		
	STAGGERED PUSH-UP (EXPLOSIVE)	30 sec.		60/30/15		
	HIGH PLANK	30 sec.		60/30/15		

heart rate	comments:
start:	
end:	
5 min. post:	

Im Athletic 6 Month Workout Plan

DATE: _____

WARM UP: CHOOSE ONE WARM FROM THE DYNAMIC FLOW DRILL LIST

		work time	KB size	rest time	reps	
Round 1	LONG CYCLE BOTTOM UP PRESS	180 sec.		90 sec.	L:	R:
	1/2 SNATCH	180 sec.		90 sec.	L:	R:
	DOUBLE SQUAT	30 sec.		60/30/15		
	BARBELL GET-UP SIT-UP	30 sec.		60/30/15		
	DOUBLE KB DEAD CLEAN	30 sec.		60/30/15		
	FIGURE 8 TO A HOLD	30 sec.		60/30/15		
	PUSH-UP	30 sec.		60/30/15		
	PLANK	30 sec.		60/30/15		

		work time	KB size	rest time	reps	
Round 2	JERK	180 sec.		90 sec.	L:	R:
	SNATCH	180 sec.		90 sec.	L:	R:
	HAND 2 HAND SUMO DEADLIFT	30 sec.		60/30/15		
	SIDE BEND (LEFT AND RIGHT)	30 sec.		60/30/15		
	ALTERNATING CLEAN (DIP & SWITCH)	30 sec.		60/30/15		
	FIGURE 8 TO A HOLD	30 sec.		60/30/15		
	CLOSE GRIP PUSH-UP (MILITARY)	30 sec.		60/30/15		

		work time	KB size	rest time	reps	
Round 3	PRESS	180 sec.		90 sec.	L:	R:
	SNATCH	180 sec.		90 sec.	L:	R:
	BEHIND THE NECK SQUAT	30 sec.		60/30/15		
	WINDMILL (LEFT AND RIGHT)	30 sec.		60/30/15		
	DOUBLE KB LONG CYCLE CLEAN	30 sec.		60/30/15		
	STAGGERED PUSH-UP (EXPLOSIVE)	30 sec.		60/30/15		
	HIGH PLANK	30 sec.		60/30/15		

heart rate	comments:
start:	
end:	
5 min. post:	

Im Athletic 6 Month Workout Plan

WARM UP: CHOOSE ONE WARM FROM THE DYNAMIC FLOW DRILL LIST

		work time	KB size	rest time	reps	
Round 1	LONG CYCLE BOTTOM UP PRESS	180 sec.		90 sec.	L:	R:
	1/2 SNATCH	180 sec.		90 sec.	L:	R:
	DOUBLE SQUAT	30 sec.		60/30/15		
	BARBELL GET-UP SIT-UP	30 sec.		60/30/15		
	DOUBLE KB DEAD CLEAN	30 sec.		60/30/15		
	FIGURE 8 TO A HOLD	30 sec.		60/30/15		
	PUSH-UP	30 sec.		60/30/15		
	PLANK	30 sec.		60/30/15		

		work time	KB size	rest time	reps	
Round 2	JERK	180 sec.		90 sec.	L:	R:
	SNATCH	180 sec.		90 sec.	L:	R:
	HAND 2 HAND SUMO DEADLIFT	30 sec.		60/30/15		
	SIDE BEND (LEFT AND RIGHT)	30 sec.		60/30/15		
	ALTERNATING CLEAN (DIP & SWITCH)	30 sec.		60/30/15		
	FIGURE 8 TO A HOLD	30 sec.		60/30/15		
	CLOSE GRIP PUSH-UP (MILITARY)	30 sec.		60/30/15		

		work time	KB size	rest time	reps	
Round 3	PRESS	180 sec.		90 sec.	L:	R:
	SNATCH	180 sec.		90 sec.	L:	R:
	BEHIND THE NECK SQUAT	30 sec.		60/30/15		
	WINDMILL (LEFT AND RIGHT)	30 sec.		60/30/15		
	DOUBLE KB LONG CYCLE CLEAN	30 sec.		60/30/15		
	STAGGERED PUSH-UP (EXPLOSIVE)	30 sec.		60/30/15		
	HIGH PLANK	30 sec.		60/30/15		

heart rate	comments:
start:	
end:	
5 min. post:	

Im Athletic 6 Month Workout Plan

DATE: _____

WARM UP: CHOOSE ONE WARM FROM THE DYNAMIC FLOW DRILL LIST

Round 1

	work time	KB size	rest time	reps	
LONG CYCLE BOTTOM UP PRESS	180 sec.		90 sec.	L:	R:
1/2 SNATCH	180 sec.		90 sec.	L:	R:
DOUBLE SQUAT	30 sec.		60/30/15		
BARBELL GET-UP SIT-UP	30 sec.		60/30/15		
DOUBLE KB DEAD CLEAN	30 sec.		60/30/15		
FIGURE 8 TO A HOLD	30 sec.		60/30/15		
PUSH-UP	30 sec.		60/30/15		
PLANK	30 sec.		60/30/15		

Round 2

	work time	KB size	rest time	reps	
JERK	180 sec.		90 sec.	L:	R:
SNATCH	180 sec.		90 sec.	L:	R:
HAND 2 HAND SUMO DEADLIFT	30 sec.		60/30/15		
SIDE BEND (LEFT AND RIGHT)	30 sec.		60/30/15		
ALTERNATING CLEAN (DIP & SWITCH)	30 sec.		60/30/15		
FIGURE 8 TO A HOLD	30 sec.		60/30/15		
CLOSE GRIP PUSH-UP (MILITARY)	30 sec.		60/30/15		

Round 3

	work time	KB size	rest time	reps	
PRESS	180 sec.		90 sec.	L:	R:
SNATCH	180 sec.		90 sec.	L:	R:
BEHIND THE NECK SQUAT	30 sec.		60/30/15		
WINDMILL (LEFT AND RIGHT)	30 sec.		60/30/15		
DOUBLE KB LONG CYCLE CLEAN	30 sec.		60/30/15		
STAGGERED PUSH-UP (EXPLOSIVE)	30 sec.		60/30/15		
HIGH PLANK	30 sec.		60/30/15		

heart rate	comments:
start:	
end:	
5 min. post:	

Im Athletic 6 Month Workout Plan

DATE: _____

WARM UP: CHOOSE ONE WARM FROM THE DYNAMIC FLOW DRILL LIST

		work time	KB size	rest time	reps	
Round 1	LONG CYCLE BOTTOM UP PRESS	180 sec.		90 sec.	L:	R:
	1/2 SNATCH	180 sec.		90 sec.	L:	R:
	DOUBLE SQUAT	30 sec.		60/30/15		
	BARBELL GET-UP SIT-UP	30 sec.		60/30/15		
	DOUBLE KB DEAD CLEAN	30 sec.		60/30/15		
	FIGURE 8 TO A HOLD	30 sec.		60/30/15		
	PUSH-UP	30 sec.		60/30/15		
	PLANK	30 sec.		60/30/15		

		work time	KB size	rest time	reps	
Round 2	JERK	180 sec.		90 sec.	L:	R:
	SNATCH	180 sec.		90 sec.	L:	R:
	HAND 2 HAND SUMO DEADLIFT	30 sec.		60/30/15		
	SIDE BEND (LEFT AND RIGHT)	30 sec.		60/30/15		
	ALTERNATING CLEAN (DIP & SWITCH)	30 sec.		60/30/15		
	FIGURE 8 TO A HOLD	30 sec.		60/30/15		
	CLOSE GRIP PUSH-UP (MILITARY)	30 sec.		60/30/15		

		work time	KB size	rest time	reps	
Round 3	PRESS	180 sec.		90 sec.	L:	R:
	SNATCH	180 sec.		90 sec.	L:	R:
	BEHIND THE NECK SQUAT	30 sec.		60/30/15		
	WINDMILL (LEFT AND RIGHT)	30 sec.		60/30/15		
	DOUBLE KB LONG CYCLE CLEAN	30 sec.		60/30/15		
	STAGGERED PUSH-UP (EXPLOSIVE)	30 sec.		60/30/15		
	HIGH PLANK	30 sec.		60/30/15		

heart rate	comments:
start:	
end:	
5 min. post:	

Im Athletic 6 Month Workout Plan

DATE: _____

WARM UP: CHOOSE ONE WARM FROM THE DYNAMIC FLOW DRILL LIST

		work time	KB size	rest time	reps	
Round 1	LONG CYCLE JERK	180 sec.		60 sec.	L:	R:
	1/2 SNATCH	180 sec.		60 sec.	L:	R:
	DOUBLE SQUAT	30 sec.		60/30/15		
	BARBELL GET-UP SIT-UP	30 sec.		60/30/15		
	DOUBLE KB DEAD CLEAN	30 sec.		60/30/15		
	FIGURE 8 TO A HOLD	30 sec.		60/30/15		
	PUSH-UP	30 sec.		60/30/15		
	PLANK	30 sec.		60/30/15		

		work time	KB size	rest time	reps	
Round 2	JERK	180 sec.		60 sec.	L:	R:
	SNATCH	180 sec.		60 sec.	L:	R:
	HAND 2 HAND SUMO DEADLIFT	30 sec.		60/30/15		
	SIDE BEND (LEFT AND RIGHT)	30 sec.		60/30/15		
	ALTERNATING CLEAN (DIP & SWITCH)	30 sec.		60/30/15		
	FIGURE 8 TO A HOLD	30 sec.		60/30/15		
	CLOSE GRIP PUSH-UP (MILITARY)	30 sec.		60/30/15		

		work time	KB size	rest time	reps	
Round 3	LONG CYCLE JERK	180 sec.		60 sec.	L:	R:
	1/2 SNATCH	180 sec.		60 sec.	L:	R:
	BEHIND THE NECK SQUAT	30 sec.		60/30/15		
	WINDMILL (LEFT AND RIGHT)	30 sec.		60/30/15		
	DOUBLE KB LONG CYCLE CLEAN	30 sec.		60/30/15		
	STAGGERED PUSH-UP (EXPLOSIVE)	30 sec.		60/30/15		
	HIGH PLANK	30 sec.		60/30/15		

heart rate	comments:
start:	
end:	
5 min. post:	

Im Athletic 6 Month Workout Plan

DATE: _____

WARM UP: CHOOSE ONE WARM FROM THE DYNAMIC FLOW DRILL LIST

Round 1

	work time	KB size	rest time	reps	
LONG CYCLE JERK	180 sec.		60 sec.	L:	R:
1/2 SNATCH	180 sec.		60 sec.	L:	R:
DOUBLE SQUAT	30 sec.		60/30/15		
BARBELL GET-UP SIT-UP	30 sec.		60/30/15		
DOUBLE KB DEAD CLEAN	30 sec.		60/30/15		
FIGURE 8 TO A HOLD	30 sec.		60/30/15		
PUSH-UP	30 sec.		60/30/15		
PLANK	30 sec.		60/30/15		

Round 2

	work time	KB size	rest time	reps	
JERK	180 sec.		60 sec.	L:	R:
SNATCH	180 sec.		60 sec.	L:	R:
HAND 2 HAND SUMO DEADLIFT	30 sec.		60/30/15		
SIDE BEND (LEFT AND RIGHT)	30 sec.		60/30/15		
ALTERNATING CLEAN (DIP & SWITCH)	30 sec.		60/30/15		
FIGURE 8 TO A HOLD	30 sec.		60/30/15		
CLOSE GRIP PUSH-UP (MILITARY)	30 sec.		60/30/15		

Round 3

	work time	KB size	rest time	reps	
LONG CYCLE JERK	180 sec.		60 sec.	L:	R:
1/2 SNATCH	180 sec.		60 sec.	L:	R:
BEHIND THE NECK SQUAT	30 sec.		60/30/15		
WINDMILL (LEFT AND RIGHT)	30 sec.		60/30/15		
DOUBLE KB LONG CYCLE CLEAN	30 sec.		60/30/15		
STAGGERED PUSH-UP (EXPLOSIVE)	30 sec.		60/30/15		
HIGH PLANK	30 sec.		60/30/15		

heart rate	comments:
start:	
end:	
5 min. post:	

Im Athletic 6 Month Workout Plan

DATE: _____

WARM UP: CHOOSE ONE WARM FROM THE DYNAMIC FLOW DRILL LIST

		work time	KB size	rest time	reps	
Round 1	LONG CYCLE JERK	180 sec.		60 sec.	L:	R:
	1/2 SNATCH	180 sec.		60 sec.	L:	R:
	DOUBLE SQUAT	30 sec.		60/30/15		
	BARBELL GET-UP SIT-UP	30 sec.		60/30/15		
	DOUBLE KB DEAD CLEAN	30 sec.		60/30/15		
	FIGURE 8 TO A HOLD	30 sec.		60/30/15		
	PUSH-UP	30 sec.		60/30/15		
	PLANK	30 sec.		60/30/15		

		work time	KB size	rest time	reps	
Round 2	JERK	180 sec.		60 sec.	L:	R:
	SNATCH	180 sec.		60 sec.	L:	R:
	HAND 2 HAND SUMO DEADLIFT	30 sec.		60/30/15		
	SIDE BEND (LEFT AND RIGHT)	30 sec.		60/30/15		
	ALTERNATING CLEAN (DIP & SWITCH)	30 sec.		60/30/15		
	FIGURE 8 TO A HOLD	30 sec.		60/30/15		
	CLOSE GRIP PUSH-UP (MILITARY)	30 sec.		60/30/15		

		work time	KB size	rest time	reps	
Round 3	LONG CYCLE JERK	180 sec.		60 sec.	L:	R:
	1/2 SNATCH	180 sec.		60 sec.	L:	R:
	BEHIND THE NECK SQUAT	30 sec.		60/30/15		
	WINDMILL (LEFT AND RIGHT)	30 sec.		60/30/15		
	DOUBLE KB LONG CYCLE CLEAN	30 sec.		60/30/15		
	STAGGERED PUSH-UP (EXPLOSIVE)	30 sec.		60/30/15		
	HIGH PLANK	30 sec.		60/30/15		

heart rate	comments:
start:	
end:	
5 min. post:	

Im Athletic 6 Month Workout Plan

WARM UP: CHOOSE ONE WARM FROM THE DYNAMIC FLOW DRILL LIST

		work time	KB size	rest time	reps	
Round 1	LONG CYCLE JERK	180 sec.		60 sec.	L:	R:
	1/2 SNATCH	180 sec.		60 sec.	L:	R:
	DOUBLE SQUAT	30 sec.		60/30/15		
	BARBELL GET-UP SIT-UP	30 sec.		60/30/15		
	DOUBLE KB DEAD CLEAN	30 sec.		60/30/15		
	FIGURE 8 TO A HOLD	30 sec.		60/30/15		
	PUSH-UP	30 sec.		60/30/15		
	PLANK	30 sec.		60/30/15		

		work time	KB size	rest time	reps	
Round 2	JERK	180 sec.		60 sec.	L:	R:
	SNATCH	180 sec.		60 sec.	L:	R:
	HAND 2 HAND SUMO DEADLIFT	30 sec.		60/30/15		
	SIDE BEND (LEFT AND RIGHT)	30 sec.		60/30/15		
	ALTERNATING CLEAN (DIP & SWITCH)	30 sec.		60/30/15		
	FIGURE 8 TO A HOLD	30 sec.		60/30/15		
	CLOSE GRIP PUSH-UP (MILITARY)	30 sec.		60/30/15		

		work time	KB size	rest time	reps	
Round 3	LONG CYCLE JERK	180 sec.		60 sec.	L:	R:
	1/2 SNATCH	180 sec.		60 sec.	L:	R:
	BEHIND THE NECK SQUAT	30 sec.		60/30/15		
	WINDMILL (LEFT AND RIGHT)	30 sec.		60/30/15		
	DOUBLE KB LONG CYCLE CLEAN	30 sec.		60/30/15		
	STAGGERED PUSH-UP (EXPLOSIVE)	30 sec.		60/30/15		
	HIGH PLANK	30 sec.		60/30/15		

heart rate	comments:
start:	
end:	
5 min. post:	

Im Athletic 6 Month Workout Plan

DATE: _____

MONTH: 6
WEEK: 4
DAY: 1

WARM UP: CHOOSE ONE WARM FROM THE DYNAMIC FLOW DRILL LIST

		work time	KB size	rest time	reps	
Round 1	PRESS	180 sec.		30 sec.	L:	R:
	SNATCH	180 sec.		30 sec.	L:	R:
	DOUBLE SQUAT	30 sec.		60/30/15		
	BARBELL GET-UP SIT-UP	30 sec.		60/30/15		
	DOUBLE KB DEAD CLEAN	30 sec.		60/30/15		
	FIGURE 8 TO A HOLD	30 sec.		60/30/15		
	PUSH-UP	30 sec.		60/30/15		
	PLANK	30 sec.		60/30/15		

		work time	KB size	rest time	reps	
Round 2	JERK	180 sec.		30 sec.	L:	R:
	SNATCH	180 sec.		30 sec.	L:	R:
	HAND 2 HAND SUMO DEADLIFT	30 sec.		60/30/15		
	SIDE BEND (LEFT AND RIGHT)	30 sec.		60/30/15		
	ALTERNATING CLEAN (DIP & SWITCH)	30 sec.		60/30/15		
	FIGURE 8 TO A HOLD	30 sec.		60/30/15		
	CLOSE GRIP PUSH-UP (MILITARY)	30 sec.		60/30/15		

		work time	KB size	rest time	reps	
Round 3	LONG CYCLE JERK	180 sec.		30 sec.	L:	R:
	SNATCH	180 sec.		30 sec.	L:	R:
	BEHIND THE NECK SQUAT	30 sec.		60/30/15		
	WINDMILL (LEFT AND RIGHT)	30 sec.		60/30/15		
	DOUBLE KB LONG CYCLE CLEAN	30 sec.		60/30/15		
	STAGGERED PUSH-UP (EXPLOSIVE)	30 sec.		60/30/15		
	HIGH PLANK	30 sec.		60/30/15		

heart rate	comments:
start:	
end:	
5 min. post:	

Im Athletic 6 Month Workout Plan

DATE: _____

WARM UP: CHOOSE ONE WARM FROM THE DYNAMIC FLOW DRILL LIST

Round 1

	work time	KB size	rest time	reps	
PRESS	180 sec.		30 sec.	L:	R:
SNATCH	180 sec.		30 sec.	L:	R:
DOUBLE SQUAT	30 sec.		60/30/15		
BARBELL GET-UP SIT-UP	30 sec.		60/30/15		
DOUBLE KB DEAD CLEAN	30 sec.		60/30/15		
FIGURE 8 TO A HOLD	30 sec.		60/30/15		
PUSH-UP	30 sec.		60/30/15		
PLANK	30 sec.		60/30/15		

Round 2

	work time	KB size	rest time	reps	
JERK	180 sec.		30 sec.	L:	R:
SNATCH	180 sec.		30 sec.	L:	R:
HAND 2 HAND SUMO DEADLIFT	30 sec.		60/30/15		
SIDE BEND (LEFT AND RIGHT)	30 sec.		60/30/15		
ALTERNATING CLEAN (DIP & SWITCH)	30 sec.		60/30/15		
FIGURE 8 TO A HOLD	30 sec.		60/30/15		
CLOSE GRIP PUSH-UP (MILITARY)	30 sec.		60/30/15		

Round 3

	work time	KB size	rest time	reps	
LONG CYCLE JERK	180 sec.		30 sec.	L:	R:
SNATCH	180 sec.		30 sec.	L:	R:
BEHIND THE NECK SQUAT	30 sec.		60/30/15		
WINDMILL (LEFT AND RIGHT)	30 sec.		60/30/15		
DOUBLE KB LONG CYCLE CLEAN	30 sec.		60/30/15		
STAGGERED PUSH-UP (EXPLOSIVE)	30 sec.		60/30/15		
HIGH PLANK	30 sec.		60/30/15		

heart rate	comments:
start:	
end:	
5 min. post:	

Im Athletic 6 Month Workout Plan

DATE: _____

WARM UP: CHOOSE ONE WARM FROM THE DYNAMIC FLOW DRILL LIST

Round 1		work time	KB size	rest time	reps	
	PRESS	180 sec.		30 sec.	L:	R:
	SNATCH	180 sec.		30 sec.	L:	R:
	DOUBLE SQUAT	30 sec.		60/30/15		
	BARBELL GET-UP SIT-UP	30 sec.		60/30/15		
	DOUBLE KB DEAD CLEAN	30 sec.		60/30/15		
	FIGURE 8 TO A HOLD	30 sec.		60/30/15		
	PUSH-UP	30 sec.		60/30/15		
	PLANK	30 sec.		60/30/15		

Round 2		work time	KB size	rest time	reps	
	JERK	180 sec.		30 sec.	L:	R:
	SNATCH	180 sec.		30 sec.	L:	R:
	HAND 2 HAND SUMO DEADLIFT	30 sec.		60/30/15		
	SIDE BEND (LEFT AND RIGHT)	30 sec.		60/30/15		
	ALTERNATING CLEAN (DIP & SWITCH)	30 sec.		60/30/15		
	FIGURE 8 TO A HOLD	30 sec.		60/30/15		
	CLOSE GRIP PUSH-UP (MILITARY)	30 sec.		60/30/15		

Round 3		work time	KB size	rest time	reps	
	LONG CYCLE JERK	180 sec.		30 sec.	L:	R:
	SNATCH	180 sec.		30 sec.	L:	R:
	BEHIND THE NECK SQUAT	30 sec.		60/30/15		
	WINDMILL (LEFT AND RIGHT)	30 sec.		60/30/15		
	DOUBLE KB LONG CYCLE CLEAN	30 sec.		60/30/15		
	STAGGERED PUSH-UP (EXPLOSIVE)	30 sec.		60/30/15		
	HIGH PLANK	30 sec.		60/30/15		

heart rate	comments:
start:	
end:	
5 min. post:	

Im Athletic 6 Month Workout Plan

DATE: _____

WARM UP: CHOOSE ONE WARM FROM THE DYNAMIC FLOW DRILL LIST

		work time	KB size	rest time	reps	
Round 1	PRESS	180 sec.		30 sec.	L:	R:
	SNATCH	180 sec.		30 sec.	L:	R:
	DOUBLE SQUAT	30 sec.		60/30/15		
	BARBELL GET-UP SIT-UP	30 sec.		60/30/15		
	DOUBLE KB DEAD CLEAN	30 sec.		60/30/15		
	FIGURE 8 TO A HOLD	30 sec.		60/30/15		
	PUSH-UP	30 sec.		60/30/15		
	PLANK	30 sec.		60/30/15		

		work time	KB size	rest time	reps	
Round 2	JERK	180 sec.		30 sec.	L:	R:
	SNATCH	180 sec.		30 sec.	L:	R:
	HAND 2 HAND SUMO DEADLIFT	30 sec.		60/30/15		
	SIDE BEND (LEFT AND RIGHT)	30 sec.		60/30/15		
	ALTERNATING CLEAN (DIP & SWITCH)	30 sec.		60/30/15		
	FIGURE 8 TO A HOLD	30 sec.		60/30/15		
	CLOSE GRIP PUSH-UP (MILITARY)	30 sec.		60/30/15		

		work time	KB size	rest time	reps	
Round 3	LONG CYCLE JERK	180 sec.		30 sec.	L:	R:
	SNATCH	180 sec.		30 sec.	L:	R:
	BEHIND THE NECK SQUAT	30 sec.		60/30/15		
	WINDMILL (LEFT AND RIGHT)	30 sec.		60/30/15		
	DOUBLE KB LONG CYCLE CLEAN	30 sec.		60/30/15		
	STAGGERED PUSH-UP (EXPLOSIVE)	30 sec.		60/30/15		
	HIGH PLANK	30 sec.		60/30/15		

heart rate	comments:
start:	
end:	
5 min. post:	

You've finished month 6!

Benefit No. 3 to Kettlebell training:

Acceleration and Deceleration training: Kettlebell drills provide intense acceleration to many of the core muscle groups such as the hips and glutes. This acceleration transfers to many athletic skills such as jumping running, and throwing. Inversely, deceleration occurs at the end of the kettlebell movement transferring that strength into your core.

Congratulations. You've come to the end of the 6 month program. By now you're no doubt stronger in body and mind.

I'm Athletic...
So are you...
We all are...

Vaughn Parker

Notes